Current State of the Art in Cysticercosis and Neurocysticercosis

Edited by Jorge Morales-Montor, Abraham Landa and Luis Ignacio Terrazas

Published in London, United Kingdom

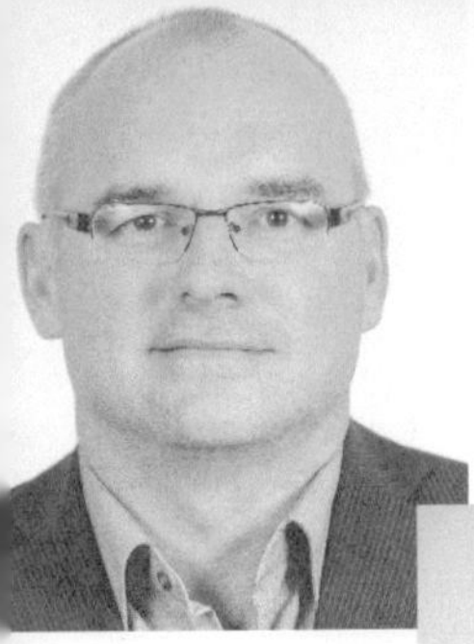
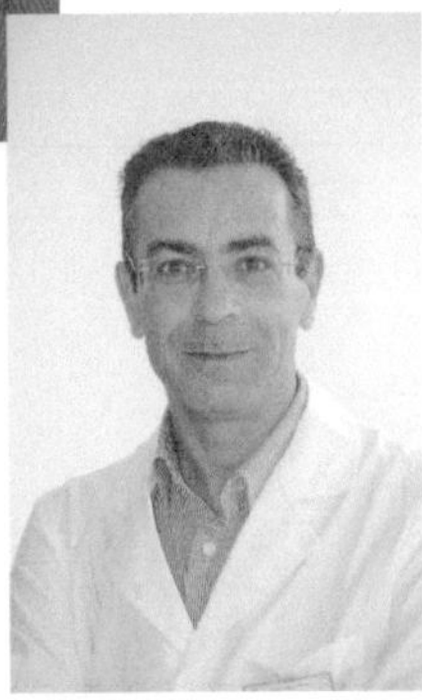
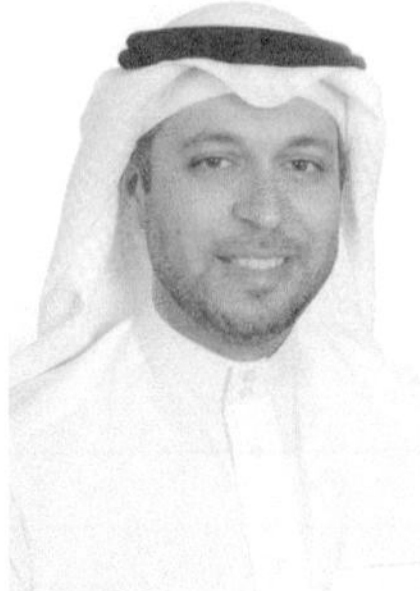
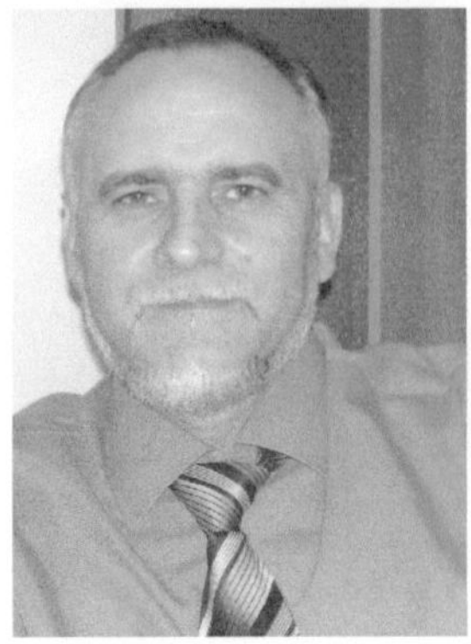
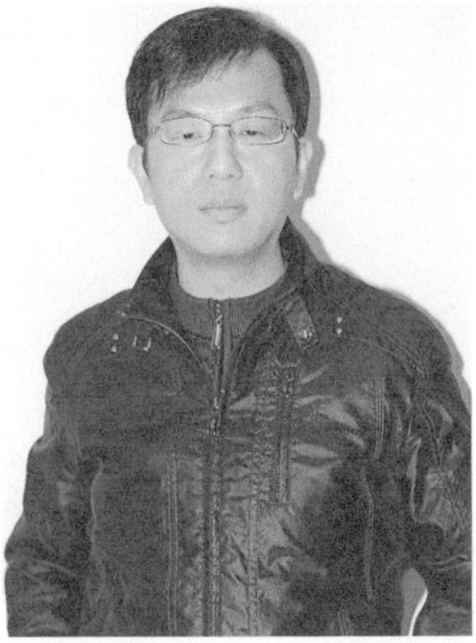
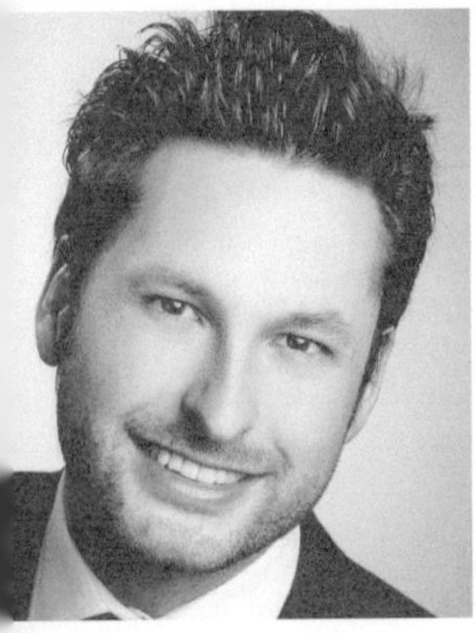
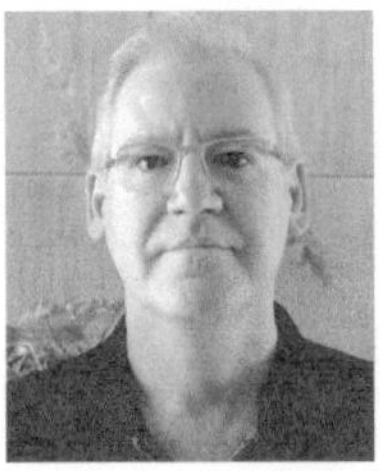

IntechOpen

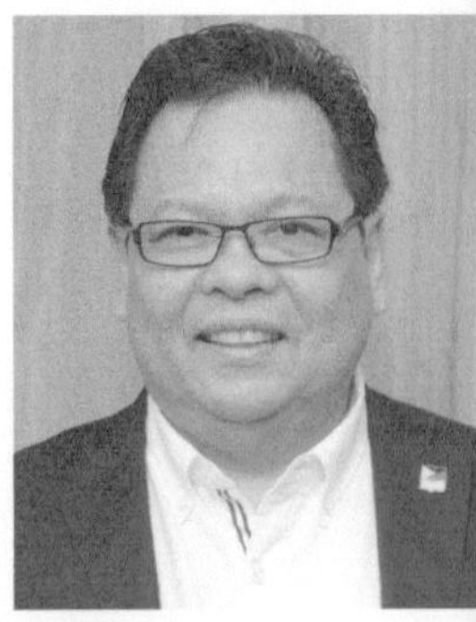
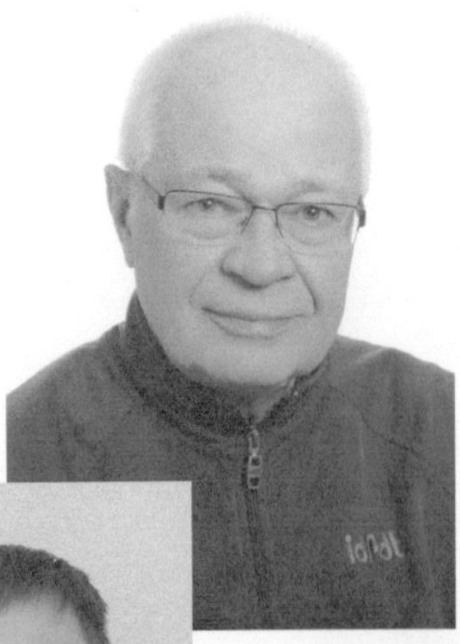
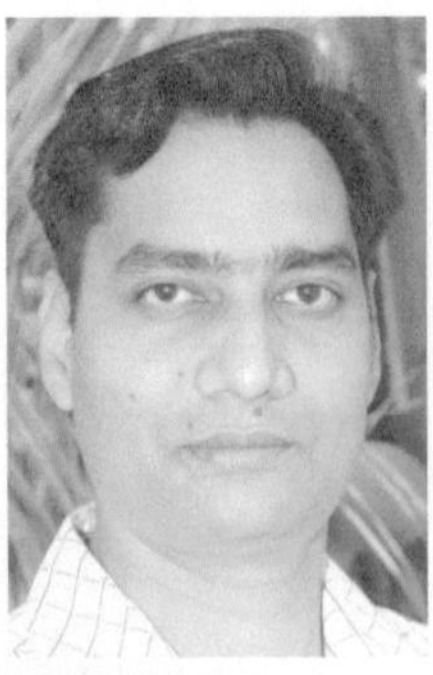
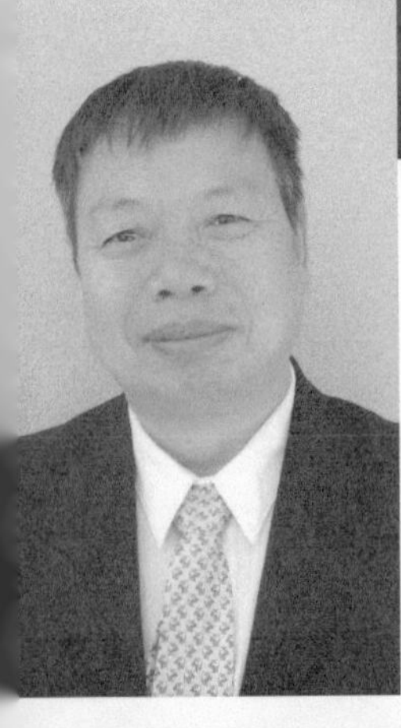
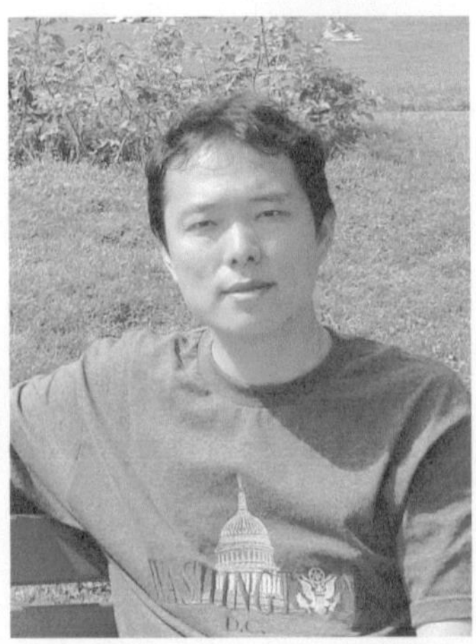
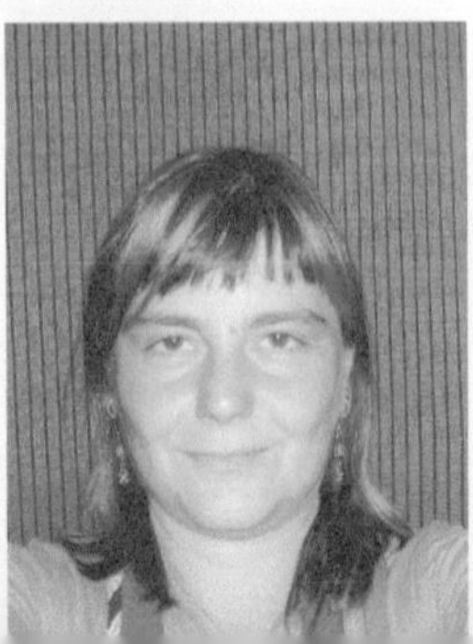

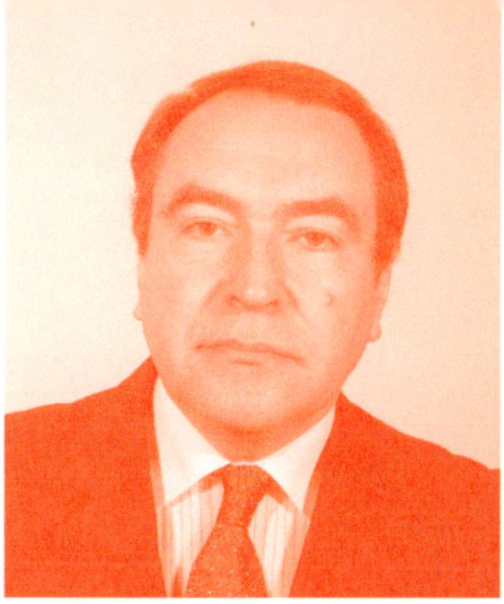

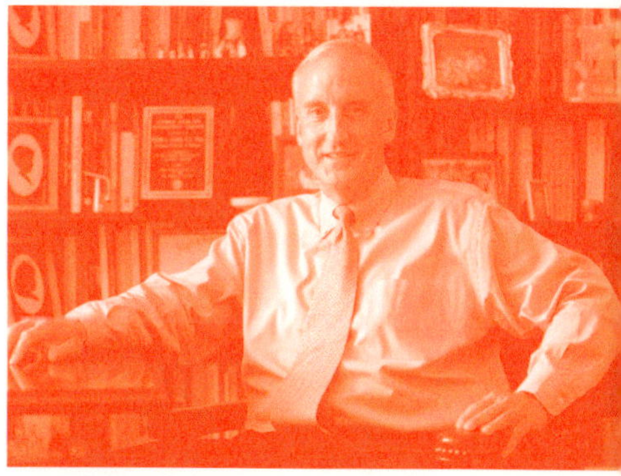

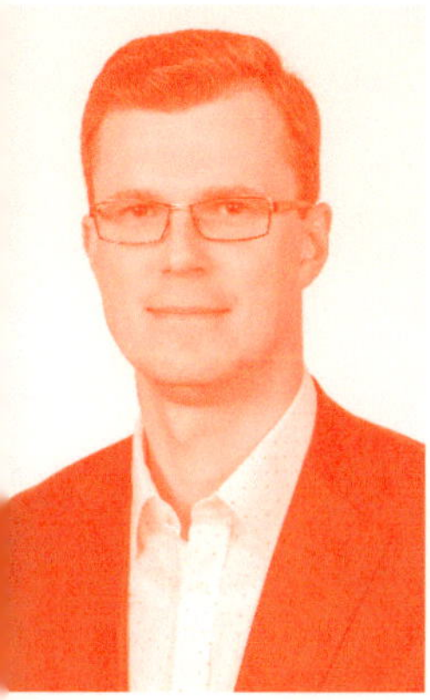

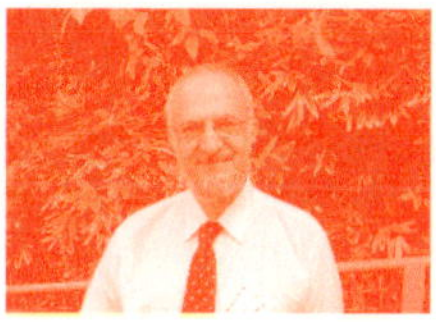

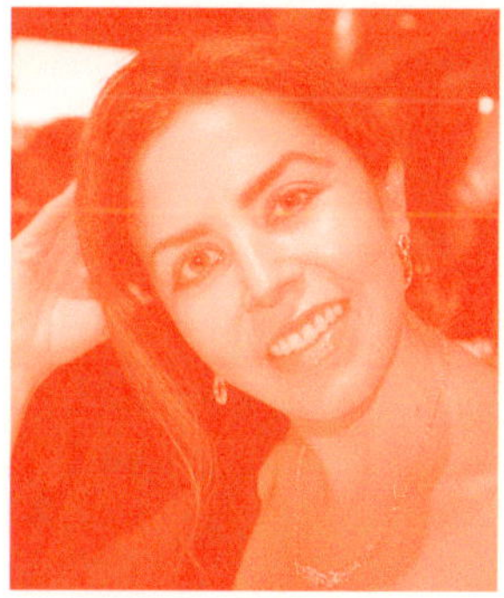

Supporting open minds since 2005

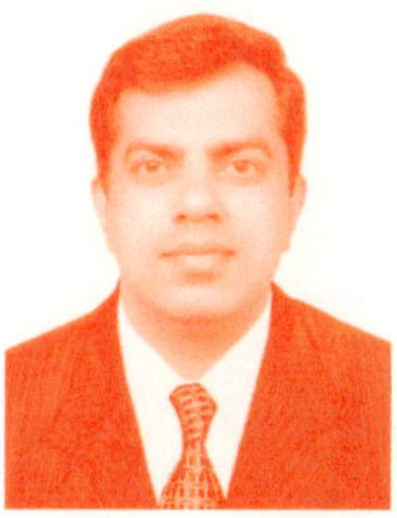

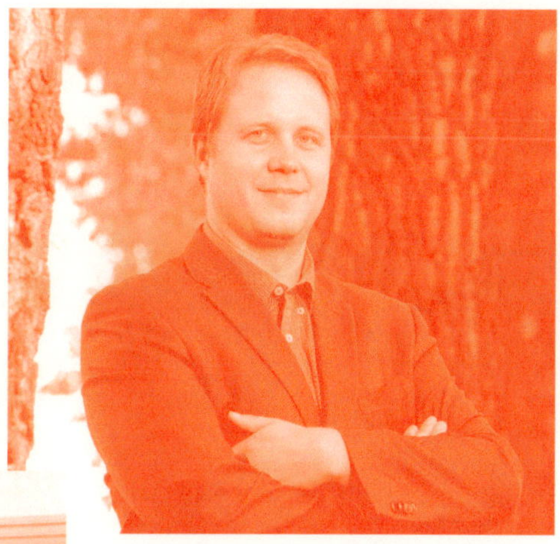

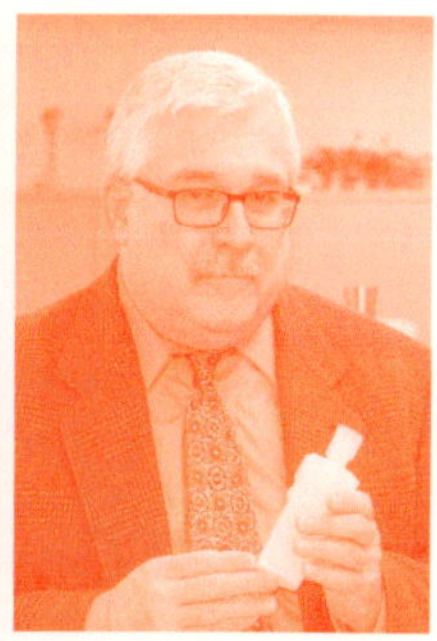

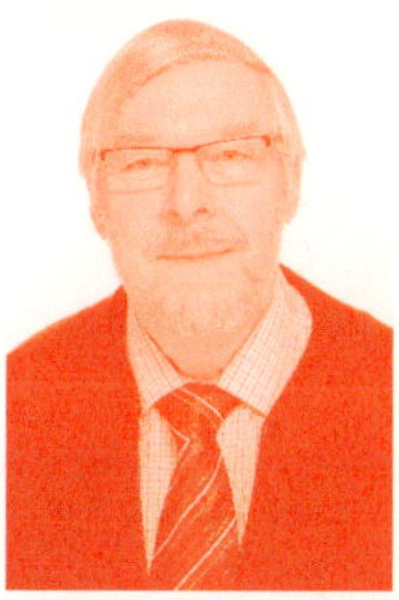

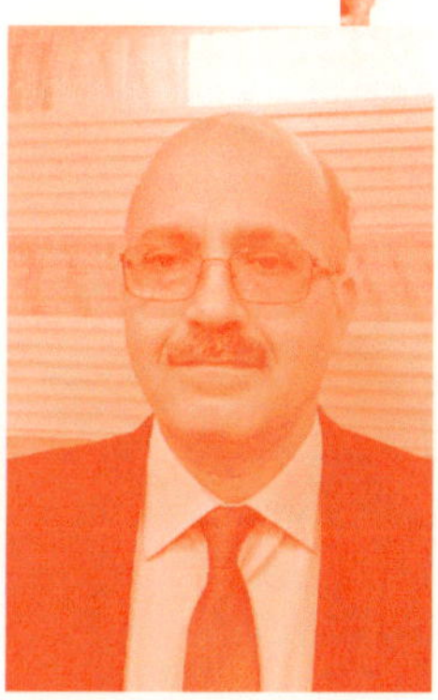

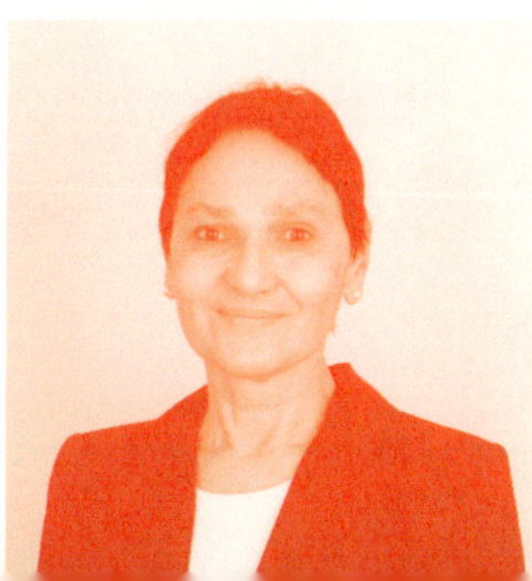

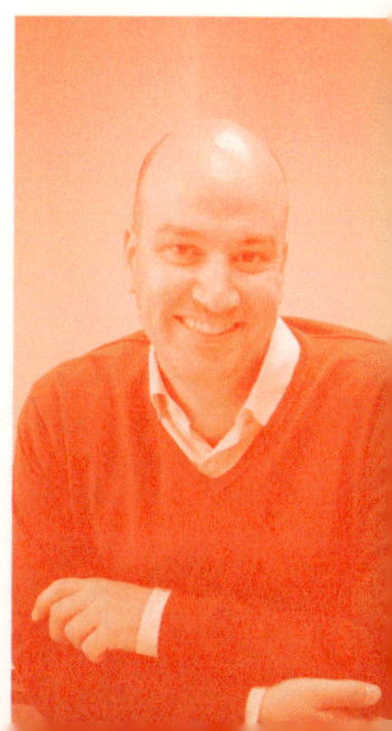

Current State of the Art in Cysticercosis and Neurocysticercosis
http://dx.doi.org/10.5772/intechopen.91540
Edited by Jorge Morales-Montor, Abraham Landa and Luis Ignacio Terrazas

Contributors
Abraham Landa, Rafael A. Zubillaga, Lucía Jiménez, Ponciano García-Gutiérrez, Marta C. Romano, Ricardo A. Valdez, Alejandra Aceves-Ramos, Martin Patricio, Pedro Jiménez, Alex I. Sánchez, Arlet Veloz, Raúl J. Bobes, Ane Karoline Medina Neri, Geraldo Bezerra Da Silva Júnior, Danielli Oliveira da Costa Lino, Ricardo Pereira Silva, Sara Da Silva Veras, Matías Gastón Pérez, Juan P. Laclette, Diana Rios-Valencia, Arturo Calderón-Gallegos, José Navarrete-Perea, Jeanette Flores-Bautista, Edda Sciutto, Marisela Hernández, Jacquelynne Cervantes, Nelly Villalobos, Cynthia Guzman, María Luis Villareal, Anabel Ortíz Caltempa, Gladis Fragoso, Jorge Morales-Montor, Marcela Esquivel-Velázquez, Carlos Larralde, Pedro Ostoa-Saloma, Víctor Hugo Del Río Araiza, Luis Ignacio Terrazas, Jonadab E. Olguín

First published in London, United Kingdom, 2021 by IntechOpen
IntechOpen is the global imprint of INTECHOPEN LIMITED, registered in England and Wales, registration number: 11086078, 5 Princes Gate Court, London, SW7 2QJ, United Kingdom
Printed in Croatia

British Library Cataloguing-in-Publication Data
A catalogue record for this book is available from the British Library

Additional hard and PDF copies can be obtained from orders@intechopen.com

Current State of the Art in Cysticercosis and Neurocysticercosis
Edited by Jorge Morales-Montor, Abraham Landa and Luis Ignacio Terrazas
p. cm.
Print ISBN 978-1-83969-394-6
Online ISBN 978-1-83969-395-3
eBook (PDF) ISBN 978-1-83969-396-0

For EU product safety concerns:
IN TECH d.o.o., Prolaz Marije Krucifikse Kozulić 3, 51000 Rijeka, Croatia, info@intechopen.com or visit our website at intechopen.com.

Meet the editors

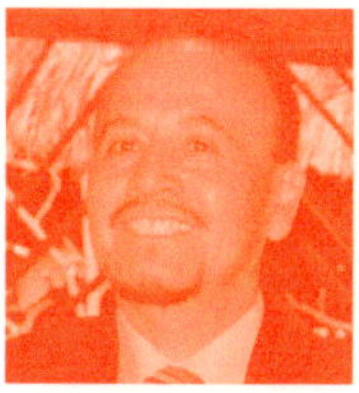

Dr. Jorge Morales-Montor was recognized with the Lola and Igo Flisser PUIS Award for best graduate thesis at the national level in the field of parasitology. He received a fellowship from the Fogarty Foundation to perform postdoctoral research stay at the University of Georgia. He has 153 journal articles to his credit. He has also edited several books and published more than fifty-five book chapters. He is a member of the Mexican Academy of Sciences, Latin American Academy of Sciences, and the National Academy of Medicine. He has received more than thirty-five awards and has supervised numerous bachelor's, master's, and Ph.D. students. Dr. Morales-Montor is the past president of the Mexican Society of Parasitology.

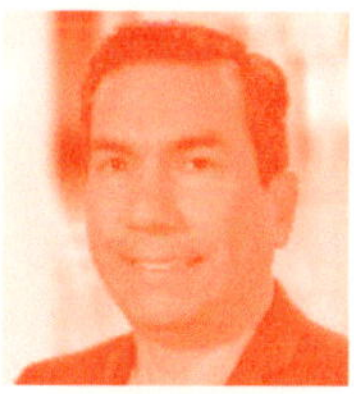

Dr. Luis Ignacio Terrazas majored in biology at Universidad Veracruzana, Mexico. He obtained a master's and a Ph.D. in Biomedical Sciences, both from the Universidad Nacional Autónoma de México (UNAM). He was a postdoctoral fellow at Harvard School of Public Health, Harvard University. He is the coordinator of the National Laboratory in Health, FES-Iztacala, UNAM. His research and career have been recognized with different awards, including first and third prizes in Basic Biomedical Sciences from the National Institutes of Health Mexico, and the State Award of Science and Technology (Biomedical Sciences) and Medal for Sciences 2016, both by the Government of the State of Mexico. He has received several travel awards from the American Association of Immunologists and the Society of Mucosal Immunity. Dr. Terrazas has more than 110 international peer-reviewed publications to his credit.

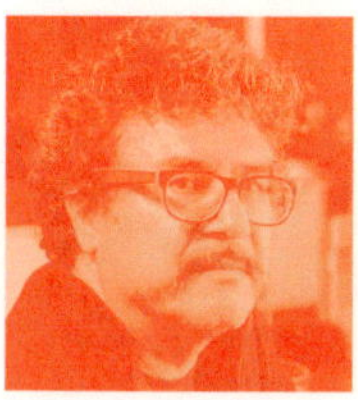

Dr. Abraham Landa obtained a BSc in Biochemistry, an MsC in Biology, and a Ph.D. in Biology, all from the Universidad Nacional Autónoma de México. He was a research fellow in the Department of Tropical Public Health, Harvard School of Public Health, Harvard University. He was awarded a second-place Lola and Igo Flisser Award for research in parasitology, the Gabino Barreda medal for his doctorate studies, and the "Nayarit for Scientific and Technological Research", awarded by the Government of Nayarit. He also was awarded a university merit award in teaching from the National Autonomous University of Mexico. He has more than seventy international peer-reviewed publications to his credit.

Contents

Preface

Cysticercosis, caused by the larval stage of *Taenia solium*, is a serious health and veterinary problem in many developing countries and is considered one of the most important neglected tropical diseases in developed countries. In humans, *T. solium* cysticerci cause neurocysticercosis, which affects approximately 50 million people worldwide and is considered an emergent disease in the United States. *T. solium* also infects pigs, its intermediate hosts, leading to major economic losses. When humans ingest undercooked contaminated pork meat, the adult worm develops in the small intestine. After two months of asymptomatic infection, this tapeworm starts producing thousands of eggs that, once released with stools, can contaminate the environment, infecting pigs (rapidly differentiating into cysticerci mainly in the muscle) and humans (where most severe symptoms are observed due to the presence of cysticerci in the brain). Thus, maintenance of the parasite's life cycle depends on the adult tapeworm development. Even in communities that do not rear or consume pigs, human neurocysticercosis can be found, because of the presence of a tapeworm carrier. Furthermore, tapeworm development depends on scolex evagination, the initial step through which a single cysticercus becomes an adult parasite with the capability of producing infective eggs. There has been a great deal of scientific advances in this field, including in vaccination, epidemiology, current drug design, diagnostics, and host-parasite interaction at all levels. However, to date, there is no book that discusses these advances in detail. As such, this book provides a comprehensive overview of the current state of the art in taeniosis/cysticercosis. It discusses recent advances in the study of cysticercosis and taeniosis, incuiding topics such as clinical disease, vaccines, immune response diagnostics, and new possible drug targets.

The book begins with a discussion in Chapter 1 by Medina Néri et al. about cardiac cysticercosis, a rare infection whose diagnosis is usually incidental because most patients are asymptomatic. Laboratory and imaging tests, such as echocardiogram and cardiac nuclear magnetic resonance, can also be used in the diagnostic approach. The clinical manifestations are broad, and patients can present with symptoms that range from heart failure to arrhythmias. Treatment of this condition has been scarcely studied and no protocols have been well established to date. One can choose not to treat the asymptomatic cases or to use cestocides, in the case of symptomatic individuals. Patient monitoring through cardiac enzymes and electrocardiogram during treatment is recommended, as well as performing imaging tests after treatment. Thus, the chapter discusses cardiac cysticercosis, covering everything from its epidemiology and clinical aspects to diagnostic methods, therapeutics, and treatment monitoring, with emphasis on the most current aspects.

In Chapter 2, Marisela Hernández et al. describe the most important advances in the development of an oral vaccine against porcine cysticercosis. Parasitic, fecally transmitted diseases, such as taeniasis/cysticercosis, represent a health problem with continued incidence due to the prevalence of inadequate sanitary conditions, particularly in developing countries. When the larval stage of the parasite is established in the central nervous system it causes neurocysticercosis, a disease that can severely affect human health. It can also cause cysticercosis in pigs, resulting in economic losses. Since pigs are obligatory intermediate hosts, they are considered targets for vaccination to interrupt the transmission of parasitosis and eventually reduce disease. Progress has been made in the development of vaccines for the prevention of porcine cysticercosis. The authors' research group identified three peptides that, when expressed synthetically (S3Pvac) or recombinantly (S3Pvac-phage), reduced the amount of cysticerci in pigs exposed to natural conditions of infection by 98.7% and 87%, respectively. Considering that cysticercosis is orally acquired, it seems feasible to develop an edible vaccine to be administered by pig farmers, simplifying the logistical difficulties of its application, reducing costs, and facilitating the implementation of vaccination programs.

In Chapter 3, Olguín et al. discuss the general differences between the different types of immunoregulation, the kind of cellular populations of the immune system used by the helminths *T. solium* and *T. crassiceps* to induce immunoregulation and immunosuppression, and the mechanisms used by these parasites such as mimicking molecules of the immune system to replace these mechanisms directly. We have learned some critical lessons about the relationship between the human body and its interaction with many infectious diseases, where the immune system has a major role in protection. We learned to differentiate between the immune response occurring in either an intracellular or extracellular parasitic infection, between innate and adaptative immune response, between either inflammatory or anti-inflammatory responses, and finally, we learned to recognize very particular mechanisms, such as the inability of the immune system to respond during certain scenarios, such as the inability of T cells to both proliferate and produce cytokines even after their exposure to mitogens or specific antigens. Along with our increased knowledge of immunology, we figured out that immunoregulation and immunosuppression are processes used by many parasites to reduce the capacity of the immune system to eliminate them, and to persist in the host favoring their transmission and completing their life cycles. Immunoregulation involves several mechanisms such as anergy, apoptosis, induction of both suppressive cytokines and membrane-bound molecules, as well as specialized cell populations of the immune system like regulatory T cells, alternatively activated macrophages, or myeloid-derived suppressor cells, which together modify the outcome of the immune response. Understanding and deciphering all these regulatory mechanisms could be useful for developing new tools to control this infection.

In Chapter 4, Esquivel-Velazquez et. al. delves into the diagnosis of neurocysticercotic patients, the complex nature of cysticercosis disease, and the simplicity of common immunological assumptions involved in explaining the low scores and reproducibility of immunotests in the diagnosis of neurocysticercosis. To begin with, the few studies dealing with the immune response during neurocysticercosis are not conclusive, which of course is crucial for developing an immunodiagnostic test. Their full recognition should clear up confusion and reduce controversy as well as provide avenues of research and technological design. In this chapter, logical arguments add that even under common immunological assumptions, serology of neurocysticercosis will always include false negative and positive results. Thus, serology is no strong support for medical diagnosis of neurocysticercosis. In contrast, immunotests performed in the cerebrospinal fluid (CSF) of neurological patients should have fewer false positives and fewer false negatives than in serum. To conclude, it is argued that high scores in serology for neurocysticercosis will not yield to usual approaches and that success needs a concerted worldwide effort. A more punctilious strategy based on the design of panels of confirmed positive and negative sera needs to be construed, shared, and tested by all interested groups to obtain comparable results. The identification of a set of specific and representative antigens of *T. solium* and a thorough compilation of the many forms of antibody response of humans to the many forms of *T. solium* disease are also to be considered as one of the most important factors to the disease.

In Chapter 5, Matías Gastón Pérez discusses the role of MicroRNAs (miRNAs) in taeniosis/cysticercosis. miRNAs are found in animals, plants, and some viruses and belong to the heterogeneous class of non-coding RNAs (ncRNAs), which post-transcriptional activity regulates gene expression. They are linked to various cellular activities such as cell growth, differentiation, development, and apoptosis. In addition, clinical trials targeting miRNAs in cancer, metabolic diseases, and viral infections have shown promising results. The chapter provides an overview of *T. solium* and *T. crassiceps* miRNAs, their possible biological functions, their role in host-parasite communication, and their potential role as biomarkers and drug targets.

In Chapter 6, Zubillaga et al. discuss the role of cytosolic glutathione transferases (GSTs) as potential drug targets. Helminth cytosolic glutathione transferases (GSTs) are essential enzymes involved in the regulation of immune responses, transport, and detoxification. In *T. solium*, three cytosolic GSTs with molecular masses of 26.5 (Ts26GST), 25.5 (Ts25GST), and 24.3 kDa (TsMσGST), classified as mu-class, mu-alpha, and sigma GST-classes, respectively, constitute the main detoxification system, and they may be immune targets for the development of vaccines and new anthelmintics. The authors performed a successful virtual screen, and identified I7, a novel selective inhibitor of Ts26GST that showed a non-competitive inhibition mechanism towards substrate glutathione with a Ki of 55.7 mM and mixed inhibition towards the electrophilic substrate 1-chloro-2,4- dinitrobenzene with a Ki of 8.64 mM. Docking simulation studies showed that I7 binds to a site adjacent to the electrophilic site and the furthest from the glutathione site. This new inhibitor of Ts26GST will be used as a lead molecule to develop new effective and safe drugs against diseases caused by *T. solium*.

In Chapter 7, Ríos-Valencia et al. discuss the post-genomic era of *T. solium* research. Cestode parasites rely on their host to obtain their nutrients. Elucidation of tapeworm genomes has shown a remarkable reduction in the coding of multiple enzymes, particularly those of anabolic pathways. Previous findings showed that 10%–13% of the proteins found in the vesicular fluid of *T. solium* cysticerci are of host origin. Further proteomic characterization allowed identification of 4,259 different proteins including 891 of host origin in the parasite's protein lysates. One explanation for this high abundance and diversity of host proteins in the parasite lysates is related to the functional exploitation of host proteins by cysticerci. Supporting this concept is the uptake of host haptoglobin and hemoglobin by the parasite as a way to acquire iron. Surprisingly, internalized host proteins are minimally degraded by the parasite's physiological machinery. Additional proteomic analysis demonstrated that these host proteins become part of the organic matrix of calcareous corpuscles as 60%–70% of the protein content is host proteins. This chapter assembles a collection of available genomic and proteomic data for taeniid cestodes and addresses the use and processing of host proteins.

Finally, in Chapter 8, Romano et al. examine the host-parasite relationship and the host's hormonal environment, which determines susceptibility to and the course and severity of several parasite infections. In most cases the infection disturbs the host environment and activates immune responses that end up affecting the endocrine system. Several reports indicate that parasites have reproductive systems, and some others have shown that these organisms synthesize sex steroid hormones. The authors show that the cysticerci of *T. crassiceps* and *T. solium* have the capacity to synthesize corticosteroids such as deoxicorticosterone and corticosterone. They also discuss the effects of thyroid hormones and infection with *T. solium* cysticerci (neurocysticercosis), and state that infection causes endocrine alterations in male and female patients.

This book assembles novel and important information about a disease that is a health burden in underdeveloped countries an emerging health problem in developed ones. We hope that readers find it a useful reference.

Jorge Morales-Montor
Departamento de Inmunología,
Instituto de Investigaciones Biomédicas,
Universidad Nacional Autónoma de México,
Ciudad de México, México

Luis Ignacio Terrazas
Unidad de Investigación Biomédica,
Facultad de Estudios Superiores Iztacala,
Universidad Nacional Autónoma de México,
Ciudad de México, México

Abraham Landa
Facultad de Medicina,
Departamento de Microbiología y Parasitología,
Universidad Nacional Autónoma de México,
Ciudad de México, México

Section 1

Clinical Cysticercosis

Chapter 1

Cardiac Cysticercosis: Current Trends in Diagnostic and Therapeutic Approaches

Ane Karoline Medina Néri,
Danielli Oliveira da Costa Lino, Sara da Silva Veras,
Ricardo Pereira Silva and Geraldo Bezerra da Silva Júnior

Abstract

Cardiac cysticercosis is a rare infection and its diagnosis is usually incidental, as most patients are asymptomatic. Laboratory and imaging tests, such as echocardiogram and cardiac nuclear magnetic resonance, can also be used in the diagnostic approach. The clinical manifestations are broad and patients can present with symptoms that range from heart failure to arrhythmias. Treatment of this condition has been scarcely studied and no protocols have been well established to date. One can choose not to treat the asymptomatic cases or to use cestocides, in the case of symptomatic individuals. Patient monitoring through cardiac enzymes and electrocardiogram during treatment is recommended, as well as performing imaging tests after treatment. This chapter aims to discuss cardiac cysticercosis, divided into sessions that will cover everything from its epidemiology and clinical aspects to diagnostic methods, therapeutics and treatment monitoring, with emphasis on the most current aspects.

Keywords: Helminthiasis, Taenia Infections, Cysticercosis, Neglected Diseases, Cysticercus, Cardiovascular Infections, Cardiac Diseases

1. Introduction

Endemic in Asia, Africa and Latin America, cysticercosis is caused by the ingestion of *Taenia solium* eggs. Contamination is caused by autoinfection in individuals with taeniasis, due to poor hand hygiene, or by heteroinfection, from contaminated foods, especially raw vegetables and water [1, 2].

The incubation period after the ingestion of the egg lasts for 3–8 weeks, with symptom onset occurring in up to 3–5 years. It is believed that the cysticercus is able to survive for a period of 3 to 6 years, after which it begins to degenerate, causing fibrosis or necrosis in the affected tissues due to the triggered inflammatory process. Nonetheless, the infection usually remains asymptomatic. Morphologically, the cysticercus exhibits two forms: the cystic form that contains the scolex and the racemous form, which corresponds to a set of vesicles, without scolex and a configuration similar to grape clusters [1].

The most affected tissues in cysticercosis are muscle and eye tissues, and the most severe manifestations are, overall, those related to the central nervous system [1].

Cardiac cysticercosis is rare, although autopsy studies have shown a 20–27% prevalence of cardiac cysticercosis occurring concomitantly with neurocysticercosis [3, 4]. In cases of cardiac involvement, pericardial effusion, signs of edema and myocardial inflammation or even myocardial infarction can occur [5].

The diagnosis can be attained by conclusively demonstrating the presence of the cysticercus through histopathological techniques in biopsy material, by visualizing the scolex in computed tomography or magnetic resonance imaging tests or by fundus examination, in cases of intraocular cysticercosis. In the absence of direct demonstration of the parasite presence, serological tests allow the diagnosis of the disease, although these tests are not widely commercially available [6].

There is no consensus on the treatment of cysticercosis with cardiac involvement. Patients with extraneural cysticercosis should be evaluated and high-risk situations, such as disseminated infections, intraventricular cysts and ocular involvement, should be excluded. Cases of asymptomatic individuals may not require surgical or anthelmintic therapy [3, 7].

The role of anthelmintics, such as Albendazole and Praziquantel, in the treatment of cardiac cysticercosis has not been directly investigated. However, it seems that the use is valid due to their effectiveness in the treatment of cysticercosis in other sites, such as neurocysticercosis. The role of cardiac surgery in the treatment of this condition also remains unclear [2].

As it is a rare condition and, therefore, still little discussed, this chapter aims to discuss the existing evidence in the literature on the diagnosis and treatment of cysticercosis with cardiac involvement, emphasizing the most current trends.

2. Epidemiology and clinical presentation of cysticercosis with cardiac involvement

Cysticercosis with cardiac involvement, especially myocardial impairment, is considered rare, and has been scarcely studied, being more frequently asymptomatic, so its diagnosis is often incidental, usually attained during cardiac surgery or at autopsy [1, 2]. Retrospective studies with autopsies have shown a variable prevalence of cardiac involvement, between 22.6% and 26.8% [3, 4, 8, 9] of the cases identified with cysticercosis.

As for the presentation according to the age group, another autopsy study showed that, of patients with cysticercosis, 27.8% were elderly and 72.2% were non-elderly, and that among the first, 20% had cardiac involvement due to cysticercosis, whereas of the latter, 25% showed cardiac cysticercosis [10]. Research [8] has shown a higher prevalence of cysticercosis in male individuals in all age groups, except for those between 30 and 39 years old, in which there was a greater number of affected women.

Cysticerci appear as oval cystic structures with thin, semitransparent and serous walls, containing liquid and measuring up to 30 mm in diameter, which contain a characteristic scolex [6]. Cysticercal involvement and distribution are variable in cardiac tissues, including the pericardium, subendocardium and myocardium [1, 6]. Cardiac cysticerci are usually multiple and, rarely, a single cardiac cyst may be present [1].

The immune system of the infected individual may not recognize the cysts for many years. However, when cysticerci age, their cystic structures can rupture, which will result in an inflammatory response [9] with variable expression and the possibility of granulomas and also fibrosis [2]. Although most cases are asymptomatic, clinical manifestations may occur as a result of inflammation, precisely at the time of spontaneous cysticercus degeneration or during treatment, which may result in different degrees of cardiac involvement [1, 2].

One study [11] showed that non-elderly individuals had significantly more cardiac inflammation than the elderly and that the inflammatory infiltrate decreases with age and depends on the evolutionary stage of the cysticercosis. Moreover, the study showed there are gender differences regarding the intensity of the inflammatory response triggered by the presence of cysticerci in the heart, with women (elderly and non-elderly) showing a more intense response to the parasitosis than men.

Therefore, in cases of cardiac involvement, myocarditis with transient left ventricular dysfunction, pericardial effusion of variable extension, restrictive cardiomyopathy due to fibrosis formation [6], ischemic heart disease [12], in addition to valve pathologies [1, 2, 6] and conduction system defects, such as bradyarrhythmia and advanced atrioventricular block [13, 14] can occur. Dilated cardiomyopathy [6] and even severe ventricular dysfunction and cardiogenic shock have also been reported, in cases with severe cardiac or cardiopulmonary infestation [15].

The reasons why some patients have multiple cysticerci, while others have a single lesion remain uncertain. In a prospective follow-up study in India with 60 patients with disseminated cysticercosis, it was observed that changes in the Toll-like receptor-4 of *Asp299Gly* and *Thr399Ile* genes increased the risk (6.63 and 4.61-fold in the presence of polymorphisms, respectively) of disseminated cysticercosis [7].

The relationship between cysticercosis and immunosuppression remains uncertain, although post-chemotherapy cases of cysticercosis have been documented in Brazil and Mexico [15, 16]. Animal experiments using chemotherapeutic drugs have suggested that innate resistance contributes to the outcome of primary infection and there is a high degree of resistance to reinfection, both in the humoral and cellular mechanisms. This resistance to reinfection is altered by immunosuppression, probably due to the delay in antibody synthesis onset [17].

Table 1 shows a summary of several cases of patients with cysticercosis and cardiac involvement reported in the literature, with patients' general characteristics, clinical manifestations and sites of disease presentation (cardiac and extracardiac).

Reference	Case report location	Patient	Presentation	Site of disease
Kalra et al. [18].	Chicago, United States of America.	35-year-old man.	Palpitations and mild shortness of breath.	Heart.
Kochanowski et al. [19].	Warsaw, Poland.	39-year-old man.	Asymptomatic.	Heart and liver.
Nery et al. [12].	Belo Horizonte, Brazil.	59-year-old man.	Angina.	Heart.
Thomas et al. [13].	Mthatha, South Africa.	42-year-old man.	Bradycardia.	Heart and brain.
Bastos et al. [20].	Belo Horizonte, Brazil.	39-year-old man.	Dyspnea, progressive low visual acuity at the left side and multiple subcutaneous nodules.	Heart, lung and brain.
Dsilva et al. [21].	Mumbai, India.	62-year-old man.	Episodes of generalized tonic–clonic seizures and multiple subcutaneous nodules over both calves, arms and nape of the neck.	Heart, brain, subcutaneous tissue, liver, and muscles.

Reference	Case report location	Patient	Presentation	Site of disease
Khandpur et al. [22].	New Delhi, India.	48-year-old man.	Innumerable soft to firm, deep-seated asymptomatic nodular swellings over the trunk and extremities.	Heart, skin, central nervous system, skeletal muscles, eye and lungs.
Vaidya et al. [23].	New Delhi, India.	27-year-old man.	Multiple subcutaneous nodules all over the patient's body.	Heart, brain, face, orbit, lungs, pancreas and spleen.
Spina et al. [6].	Sydney, Australia.	24-year-old woman.	Frontal headaches, high fever, sweating, arthralgia, nausea, vomiting and weight loss of about 6 kg in one month.	Heart, brain, pancreas, liver, pleura and skeletal muscles.
Jain et al. [24].	Mumbai, India.	19-year-old man.	Headache and vomiting, seizures, decreased vision and bilateral proptosis.	Heart, brain, extradural spinal space, muscles, lungs, pancreas, and eyes.
Eberly et al. [25].	De Bilt, The Netherlands.	17-year-old boy.	Asymptomatic.	Heart.
Sousa et al. [26].	Fortaleza, Brazil.	26-year-old man.	Headache and generalized seizures.	Heart, brain and subcutaneous tissue.
Melo et al. [27].	Salvador, Brazil.	46-year-old woman.	Dyspnea on exertion and palpitations.	Heart, brain and muscles.
Mauad et al. [15].	São Paulo, Brazil.	53-year-old woman.	Mental confusion, incoherent speech and hypoactive behavior.	Heart, lungs, pleura, subcutaneous tissue and brain.
Robinson et al. [28].	Montreal, Canada.	33-year-old man.	Skin nodules, polyarthritis, hemolytic anemia, and malnutrition.	Heart, skin, muscles, brain, larynx, pleura and liver.
Sun et al. [14].	Beijing, People's Republic of China.	33-year-old man.	Headache, nausea, vomiting, and bradycardia.	Heart, brain and subcutaneous tissue.

Table 1.
Clinical characteristics, sites of disease presentation (cardiac and extracardiac), and clinical manifestations in patients reported in the literature.

3. Current diagnostic and therapeutic approaches to cardiac cysticercosis

3.1 Diagnostic methods used in the analysis of cardiac involvement due to cysticercosis

The diagnosis of cardiac cysticercosis can be attained by conclusively demonstrating the presence of the cysticercus through histopathological techniques in biopsy material or by visualizing the scolex, either by computed tomography or nuclear magnetic resonance imaging tests. Some authors consider these tests to be the gold standard in the diagnosis of cysticercosis, as they allow the visualization of the parasite and the host's reaction process [29].

The computed tomography shows greater sensitivity in the detection of calcified cysticerci, whereas the magnetic resonance imaging has greater resolution power, which may show the scolex with better accuracy [6, 30]. The echocardiogram may play a role in identifying cardiac cysts and occasionally identifies cysts consistent with cysticercosis during routine screening for other purposes [1, 6].

In the absence of direct visualization of the parasite, serological tests allow the disease diagnosis [1, 6, 30, 31]. The oldest tests, which used unfractionated antigens, including the enzyme-linked immunosorbent assay (ELISA), have been associated with high rates of false-positive and false-negative reactions [21, 30]. Currently, the Enzyme-linked immunoelectrotransfer blot (EITB) is considered one of the most reliable immunological tests for the diagnosis of cysticercosis and neurocysticercosis [29, 31]. The initial evaluation of this test indicates a 98% sensitivity and 100% specificity in serum and cerebrospinal fluid (CSF) samples. Other studies have reported an 86–100% variation in sensitivity in serum and 81–100% in CSF, while the variation in specificity ranged from 93–100% in both sample types [29]. Unfortunately, the availability of these tests is experimental, not being commercially available and rarely available at most medical centers, except for research centers working in this area [31].

Some laboratory alterations can be identified in cardiac cysticercosis, such as marked peripheral eosinophilia disclosed in the blood count, albeit only in the case of a ruptured cyst [1, 32]. Most individuals affected by this pathology do not have viable *Taenia solium* in the intestine, making the stool parasitological test ineffective [1, 31, 32].

Figure 1 summarizes the main diagnostic methods that can be used for the diagnostic definition of cysticercosis with cardiac involvement.

3.2 Treatment and monitoring of the patient with cysticercosis and cardiac involvement

There is no consensus regarding the treatment of cardiac cysticercosis. In patients with extra-neural cysticercosis, the existence of high-risk conditions, such as disseminated infection, intraventricular cysts and ocular involvement, should be evaluated [1, 31]. Asymptomatic cases might not require more specific

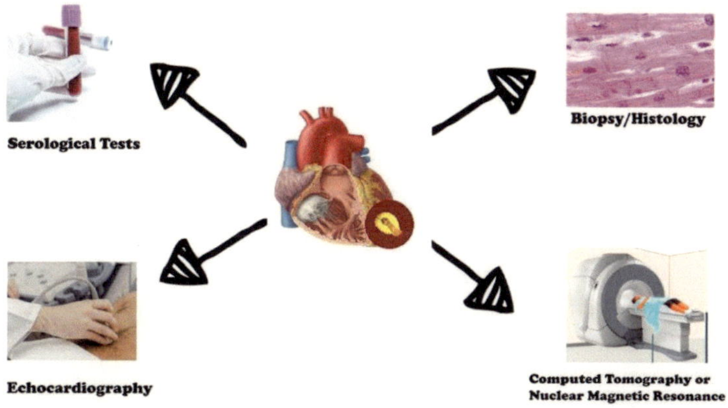

Figure 1.
Diagnostic methods that can be used for the diagnostic definition of cysticercosis with cardiac involvement.

Reference	Cardiac manifestations	Diagnostic methods	Cardiac structures involved	Treatments performed	Course of disease
Kalra et al. [18].	Palpitations and mild shortness of breath.	Magnetic resonance and serological tests by Western blot.	Anterior wall of the left ventricle.	Oral Albendazole 400 mg twice a day for 2 weeks.	One week after completing the treatment a repeat cardiac magnetic resonance showed that the lesion had decreased considerably in size.
Kochanowski et al. [19].	None.	Magnetic resonance, computed tomography and specific antibodies in serum.	Apical segment of the anterior left ventricular wall.	No specific treatment was performed.	The patient has been followed for 16 years and has had no cardiac symptoms.
Nery et al. [12].	Angina, new 1-mm ST-segment elevation of the inferior and lateral walls, and elevated cardiac troponin level.	Echocardiography, magnetic resonance and biopsy of the cardiac mass.	Intramural lesion at the left ventricular apex with extension through the free wall into the pericardial space.	Cardiac surgery. Specific drugs for the treatment of cysticercosis were not prescribed.	The postoperative period was uneventful, and the patient was discharged on day 6 postoperatively. The patient was symptom free at follow-up.
Thomas et al. [13].	Bradycardia and complete heart block.	Computed tomography and echocardiography.	The exact location of the lesions was not described, although it was reported that there were multiple myocardial calcified and active cysts.	Treatment was started only with Prednisolone (there is no description on dose and treatment duration with this drug), and five days later with the anti-helminthic drug (Praziquantel 50 mg/kg/day for 14 days).	Repeat electrocardiogram after a week of treatment showed sinus rhythm with a heart rate of 70 beats per minute.
Bastos et al. [20].	Dyspnea.	Computed tomography and an excisional biopsy of a subcutaneous nodule.	Myocardium (the exact location of the cysticercus was not described).	Albendazole (there is no description regarding the dose, route of administration and treatment duration).	Two months later the chest radiographies were normal and the patient was asymptomatic.
Dsilva et al. [21].	None.	Nuclear magnetic resonance.	Ventricular myocardium and right pericardial fat pad.	Patient was started on Albendazole 15 mg/kg/day, divided in two doses and Prednisolone 1 mg/kg in tapering doses along with Phenytoin for 28 days.	There is no description of the evolution of cardiac lesions. A review brain nuclear magnetic resonance with whole body screening was performed after treatment completion, which showed a reduction in the number of active lesions.

DOI: http://dx.doi.org/10.5772/intechopen.97472

Reference	Cardiac manifestations	Diagnostic methods	Cardiac structures involved	Treatments performed	Course of disease
Khandpur et al. [22].	None.	Computed tomography, echocardiography and skin biopsy.	Anterior cardiac wall.	Specific drugs for the treatment of cysticercosis were not prescribed. Carbamazepine 200 mg twice daily was used for seizure prevention.	The patient is still being followed by the medical team and is well.
Vaidya et al. [23].	None.	Computed tomography and anticysticercal antibodies by enzyme-linked immunosorbent assay (ELISA).	Interventricular septum musculature.	Patient was treated with oral Albendazole and antiepileptic medication. There is no description of the administered doses or treatment duration	The patient showed good evolution and was discharged with instructions to maintain regular follow-ups.
Spina et al. [6].	Tachycardia, hypotension, respiratory distress, pleuritic chest discomfort and large pericardial effusion.	Magnetic resonance and serological test for the presence of cysticerci in serum and cerebrospinal fluid.	Multiple myocardial and epicardial cysts in the left ventricular anterior, septal, posterior and lateral walls.	Prednisone (1 mg/kg daily), followed by 15 days of Albendazole (400 mg twice daily).	A repeat cardiac magnetic resonance after 9 months showed resolution of the myocardial cysts, pericardial effusion, and myocardial inflammation. On follow-up one year later, the patient was well.
Jain et al. [24].	None.	Magnetic resonance, echocardiography, muscle biopsy.	Cardiac muscle.	Specific drugs used for the treatment of Cysticercosis were not prescribed. The patient was treated symptomatically with antiepileptic drugs, steroids, and diuretics.	There is no description regarding patient evolution and follow-up.
Eberly et al. [25].	None.	Computed tomography, nuclear magnetic resonance and biopsy.	Left ventricle along the endocardial surface of the anterior wall near the anteroseptal basal region.	Cardiac surgery and one-month course of Albendazole (daily dose and route of administration were not reported).	The patient's postoperative course was uneventful. A follow-up echocardiography one month later was normal.
Sousa et al. [26].	Acute heart failure and shock.	Subcutaneous nodule biopsy, computed tomography and echocardiography.	The location of the cardiac cysticerci was not described.	Patient was treated with Phenytoin, Diazepam, Dexamethasone and Thiabendazole. There was no information on doses, administration routes or treatment duration.	One year after discharge, the patient was doing well taking only Phenytoin.

Reference	Cardiac manifestations	Diagnostic methods	Cardiac structures involved	Treatments performed	Course of disease
Melo et al. [27].	Left ventricular (LV) overload, secondary alterations in ventricular repolarization, supraventricular ectopic activity and LV diastolic dysfunction.	Positive hemagglutination reaction up to 1: 4 for cerebrospinal cysticercosis and ELISA reaction for positive anti-*Cysticercus cellulosae* antibody detection. Microcalcifications were also shown on the transthoracic echocardiography, a pattern similar to that demonstrated in plain soft tissue radiography.	Diffuse myocardial microcalcifications in both ventricles.	No treatment was carried out with antiparasitic agents.	The patient showed evolution with significant clinical improvement after specific treatment for restrictive cardiomyopathy, being referred for outpatient treatment with a cardiologist.
Mauad et al. [15] .	Acute heart failure and shock.	Patient died before diagnosis was attained.	Subendocardium, subpericardium and in-tramyocardium.	No specific treatment was implemented.	Patient died during hospitalization.
Robinson et al. [28].	Pericardial effusion, large left ventricular apical filling defect and severe tricuspid stenosis.	There is no description of the diagnostic methods.	Epicardium, myocardium (left ventricular apex), inferior vena cava, tricuspid valve and pulmonary artery.	Cardiac surgery and pharmacological treatment (drugs used in the treatment were not described).	Unstable postoperative course, requiring inotropic support and intra-aortic balloon pump. Patient died eleven weeks postoperatively.
Sun et al. [14].	Complete intra-Hisian block.	Subcutaneous nodule biopsy and complement fixation test for *Cysticercus cellulosae*.	The cardiac location of the cysticercus was not described.	The patient was treated with Mannitol and Furosemide and then with Praziquantel. There is no description regarding the dose, route of administration and treatment duration with these drugs.	The subcutaneous nodules decreased in size and the symptoms due to increased intracranial pressure disappeared, but complete AV block persisted. The patient refused a pacemaker implantation.

Table 2.
Diagnostic methods and treatments used, evolution and course of the disease in cases of cysticercosis with cardiac involvement reported in the literature.

therapy, such as surgical procedures or anthelmintic pharmacological therapy [3, 7]. In cases of asymptomatic myocardial involvement, there is usually no justification for any type of intervention, given the benign prognosis associated with this condition [3, 6].

The role of anthelmintic drugs such as Albendazole and Praziquantel in the treatment of cardiac cysticercosis has not been directly investigated in large studies; however, it seems that their use is valid due to their efficacy in the treatment of cysticercosis in other sites, such as neurocysticercosis [6]. Therefore, these drugs are used at the same dose and duration utilized to treat neurocysticercosis, with Praziquantel at a dose of 50 mg/kg/day for 15 days and Albendazole at a dose of 15 mg/kg/day for 8–15 days [6, 30, 31]. In case of a solitary cyst or granuloma, monotherapy with Albendazole may be sufficient [31].

The role of the surgical removal of cysts through cardiac surgery for the treatment of cardiac cysticercosis is also not yet clear and may be indicated when some valvular apparatus is compromised, when there is left ventricular outflow tract obstruction or even when there is epicardial coronary artery compression, with subsequent myocardial blood supply reduction [6, 12, 25, 28].

Corticosteroids are used together with antiparasitic agents in the initial treatment of neurocysticercosis to decrease the pericystic inflammatory reaction that follows larval necrosis, but there is no definition regarding its use in patients with cardiac involvement, although it is theoretically possible [1, 2, 7, 17]. A randomized trial comparing 6 mg/day of Dexamethasone for 10 days with 8 mg/day for 28 days, followed by a gradual reduction over 2 weeks, suggested that increasing the dose of Dexamethasone results in fewer seizures during treatment for neurocysticercosis [30, 31]. However, in some cardiac conditions, such as pericarditis, steroids have been associated with increased relapse and recurrence. Due to the rapid response to anti-helminthic therapy in some cases, Albendazole can be used without steroids, but with adequate monitoring [18].

Cardiac monitoring is recommended, with cardiac enzymes and electrocardiogram, during the early stages of the treatment for cardiac impairment due to cysticercosis [6]. The cases reported in the literature show that the lesions on the MRI disappear 6 to 9 months after treatment [1, 16]. However, there is no recommendation on the most appropriate periodicity for the assessment of myocardial necrosis biomarkers, or imaging tests after treatment [6].

Table 2 shows a summary of several cases reported in the literature regarding compromised cardiac structures, the several methods used for the diagnosis, the performed treatments and their monitoring, in addition to the disease evolution in each case of cysticercosis with reported cardiac impairment.

4. Conclusion

The clinical management of cysticercosis with cardiac involvement is complex, due to the rarity of the pathology and the broad spectrum of clinical presentation, ranging from asymptomatic cases to those with more severe manifestations, such as cardiogenic shock and advanced cardiac blocks. The lack of studies directly investigating the role of diagnostic methods for its detection, as well as drug therapy effectiveness with anthelmintic drugs and corticosteroids, and the role of the surgical approach are also factors that have an impact on the management of these cases. Therefore, we propose that individuals with cardiac cysticercosis should be evaluated individually by a multidisciplinary team, so that the best diagnostic and therapeutic conduct, as well as the best way of monitoring each specific case, can be implemented.

Acknowledgements

We would like to thank the Brazilian Research Council (Conselho Nacional de Desenvolvimento Científico e Tecnológico – CNPq) for supporting our research (research grant to GBSJ # 310974/2020-8).

Conflicts of interest

The authors declare no conflicts of interest.

Author details

Ane Karoline Medina Néri[1,2,3*], Danielli Oliveira da Costa Lino[1], Sara da Silva Veras[4], Ricardo Pereira Silva[3,5] and Geraldo Bezerra da Silva Júnior[1,2]

1 Postgraduate Program in Collective Health, Health Sciences Center, University of Fortaleza, Fortaleza, Ceará, Brazil

2 School of Medicine, University of Fortaleza, Fortaleza, Ceará, Brazil

3 Cardiology Service, Walter Cantídio Teaching Hospital, School of Medicine, Federal University of Ceará, Fortaleza, Ceará, Brazil

4 Infectious Diseases Service, Walter Cantídio Teaching Hospital, School of Medicine, Federal University of Ceará, Fortaleza, Ceará, Brazil

5 Postgraduate Program in Cardiovascular Sciences, Department of Clinical Medicine, School of Medicine, Federal University of Ceará, Fortaleza, Ceará, Brazil

*Address all correspondence to: karolinemedina@gmail.com

References

[1] Hidron A, Vogenthaler n, Santos-Preciado JI, Rodriguez-Morales AJ, Franco-Paredes C, Rassi A Jr. Cardiac Involvement with parasitic infections. Clin Microbiol Rev. 2010;23(2):324-349. DOI: 10.1128/CMR.00054-09

[2] Groom Z, Protopapas AD, Zochios V. Tropical diseases of the myocardium: a review. Int J Gen Med. 2017;10:101-111. DOI: https://doi.org/10.2147/IJGM.S130828

[3] Lino RSA Jr, Reis MA, Teixeira VPA. Occurrence of encephalic and cardiac cysticercosis (Cysticercus cellulosae) in necropsy. Rev Saúde Pública. 1999;33(5):495-498. DOI: https://doi.org/10.1590/S0034-89101999000500009

[4] Gobbi H, Adad SJ, Neves RR, Almeida HO. Ocorrência de cisticercose (Cysticercus cellulosae) em pacientes necropsiados em Uberaba, MG. Rev Patol Trop. 1980;9(1):51-59. DOI: https://doi.org/10.5216/rpt.v9i1%20e%202.21345

[5] Beyersdorf F, Rylski B. Cysticercosis-rare but important. J Thorac Cardiovasc Surg. 2018;155(5):e159. DOI: https://doi.org/10.1016/j.jtcvs.2017.10.104

[6] Spina R, Sandaradura I, Puranik R, Lee AS. Cardiac cysticercosis. Int J Cardiol. 2013;168(1):557-559. DOI: https://doi.org/10.1016/j.ijcard.2013.01.183

[7] Qavi A, Garg RK, Malhotra HS, Jain A, Kumar N, Malhotra KP, et al. Disseminated cysticercosis. Medicine. 2016;95(39):e4882. DOI: 10.1097/md.0000000000004882

[8] Costa-Cruz JM, Rocha A, Silva AM, Moraes AT, Guimarães AHB, Salomão EC, et al. Occurrence of cysticercosis in autopsies perfomed in Uberlândia, Minas Gerais, Brazil. Arq Neuro-Psiquiatr. 1995;53(2):227-232. DOI: https://doi.org/10.1590/S0004-282X1995000200007

[9] Franco-Paredes C, Rouphael N, Méndez J, Folch E, Rodríguez-Morales AJ, Santos JI, et al. Cardiac manifestations of parasitic infections part 3: pericardial and miscellaneous cardiopulmonary manifestations. Clin Cardiol. 2007;30(6):277-280. DOI: https://doi.org/10.1002/clc.20092

[10] Cavellani CL, Faleiros ACG, Lino RSA Jr, Reis MA, Teixeira VPA. Cysticercosis in the elderly. Ann Diagn Pathol. 2007;11(5):330-333. DOI: https://doi.org/10.1016/j.anndiagpath.2006.12.008

[11] Cavellani CL, Corrêa RRM, Ferraz MLF, Rocha LP, Faleiros ACG, Lino RSA Jr, Reis MA, Teixeira VPA. Influence of gender on cardiac and encephalic inflammation in the elderly with cysticercosis: a case control study. J Trop Med. 2012;2012. DOI: https://doi.org/10.1155/2012/540858

[12] Nery TB, Gelape CL, Passaglia LG, Carmo GAL. Cardiac cysticercosis: a rare cause of myocardial infarction. J Thorac Cardiovasc Surg. 2018;155(5):155-158. DOI: https://doi.org/10.1016/j.jtcvs.2017.10.058

[13] Thomas MB, Thomas KM, Awotedu AA, Blanco-Blanco E, Anwary M. Cardiocysticercosis. S Afr Med J. 2007;97(7):504-505. Available from: http://www.samj.org.za/index.php/samj/article/view/594/119 [Accessed: 16 November 2020]

[14] Sun RL, Wang FZ, Hu SJ, Tian RG. Intra-Hisian block associated with unusual etiologies. Chin Med J (Engl). 1987;100(3):167-172. DOI: https://doi.org/10.1111/j.1540-8159.1987.tb06130.x

[15] Mauad T, Battlehner CN, Bedrikow CL, Capelozzi VL,

Saldiva PH. Case report: massive cardiopulmonary cysticercosis in a leukemic patient. Pathol Res Pract. 1997;193(7):527-529. DOI: https://doi.org/10.1016/S0344-0338(97)80108-2

[16] Sanz CR. Host response in childhood neurocysticercosis. Child's Nerv Syst. 1987;3(4):206-207. DOI: https://doi.org/10.1007/BF00274046

[17] Bojalil R, Terrazas LI, Govezensky T, Sciutto E, Larralde C. Thymus-related cellular immune mechanisms in sex-associated resistance to experimental murine cysticercosis (Taenia crassiceps). J Parasitol. 1993;79(3): 384-389. DOI: https://doi.org/10.2307/3283574

[18] Kalra DK, Rao A, Simms A, Pierre-Louis A. Isolated cardiac cysticercosis: treatment with or without steroids? Lancet. 2019;393(10189):2439. DOI: https://doi.org/10.1016/S0140-6736(19)31268-1

[19] Kochanowski J, Budnik M, Odyniec-Nowacka M, Opolski G. Unusual mass in the left ventricle. Circ J. 2019;83(2):488. DOI https://doi.org/10.1253/circj.CJ-17-1301

[20] Bastos AL, Marchiori E, Gasparetto EL, Andrade BH, Junior GC, Carvalho RC, et al. Pulmonary and cardiac cysticercosis: helical CT findings. Br J Radiol. 2007;80(951):58-60. DOI: https://doi.org/10.1259/bjr/43104295

[21] Dsilva G, Kulkarni V, Aher S. An uncommon manifestation of a common disease. Ann Parasitol. 2017;63(4):357-360. DOI: 10.17420/ap6304.124

[22] Khandpur S, Kothiwala SK, Basnet B, Nangia R, Venkatesh HA, Sharma R. Extensive disseminated cysticercosis. Indian J Dermatol Venereol Leprol. 2014;80(2):137-140. DOI: 10.4103/0378-6323.129389

[23] Vaidya A. Asymptomatic disseminated cysticercosis. J Clin Diagn Res. 2013;7(8):1761-1763. DOI: 10.7860/JCDR/2013/5465.3269

[24] Jain B, Sankhe S, Agrawal M, Naphade P. Disseminated cysticercosis with pulmonary and cardiac involvement. Indian J Radiol Imaging. 2010;20(4):310-313. DOI: 10.4103/0971-3026.73532

[25] Eberly MD, Soh EK, Bannister SP, Tavaf-Motamen H, Scott JS. Isolated cardiac cysticercosis in an adolescent. Pediatr Infect Dis J. 2008;27(4):369-371. DOI: 10.1097/INF.0b013e318163d316

[26] Sousa AQ, Solon FRN, Costa Filho JE, Lima FHC. Disseminated cysticercosis with asymptomatic involvement of the heart. Braz J Infect Dis. 2006;10(1):65. DOI: http://dx.doi.org/10.1590/S1413-86702006000100014

[27] Melo RMV, Melo Neto AV, Corrêa LCL, Melo Filho AV. Cardiomiopatia restritiva por cisticercose miocárdica. Arq Bras Cardiol. 2005;85(6):425-427. DOI: http://dx.doi.org/10.1590/S0066-782X2005001900009

[28] Robinson RJ, Truong DT, Mulder D, Digerness SB, Kirklin JK. Case 1989-3. A 33-year-old woman develops a "stone heart" and is successfully treated with magnesium. J Cardiothorac Anesth. 1989;3(3):361-368. DOI: 10.1016/0888-6296(89)90122-1

[29] Togoro SY, Souza EM, Sato NS. Laboratory diagnosis of neurocysticercosis: review and perspectives. J Bras Patol Med Lab. 2012;48(5):345-355. DOI: https://doi.org/10.1590/S1676-24442012000500007

[30] White AC Jr. Neurocysticercosis: updates on epidemiology, pathogenesis, diagnosis, and management. Annu Rev

Med. 2000;51:187-206. DOI: https://doi.org/10.1146/annurev.med.51.1.187

[31] Zammarchi L, Bonati M, Strohmeyer M, Albonico M, Requena-Méndez A, Bisoffi Z, et al. Screening, diagnosis and management of human cysticercosis and Taenia soliumtaeniasis: technical recommendations by the cohemi project study group. Trop Med Int Health. 2017;22(7):881-894. DOI: https://doi.org/10.1111/tmi.12887

[32] Takayanagui OM. Cisticercose. In: Tavares W, organizador. Rotinas de diagnóstico e tratamento das doenças infecciosas e parasitárias. 4ª ed. São Paulo: Atheneu, 2015. p. 179-184.

Section 2

Recent Advances in Cysticercosis Research: Vaccine Immune Response and Immunodiagnosis

Chapter 2

Development of an Oral Vaccine for the Control of Cysticercosis

Marisela Hernández, Anabel Ortiz Caltempa, Jacquelynne Cervantes, Nelly Villalobos, Cynthia Guzmán, Gladis Fragoso, Edda Sciutto and María Luisa Villareal

Abstract

Parasitic diseases fecally transmitted, such taeniasis/cysticercosis *Taenia solium* binomial, represent a health problem whose incidence continues due to the prevalence of inadequate sanitary conditions, particularly in developing countries. When the larval stage of the parasite is established in the central nervous system causes neurocysticercosis a disease than can severely affect human health. It can also affect pigs causing cysticercosis causing economic losses. Since pigs are obligatory intermediate hosts, they have been considered as the targets for vaccination to interrupt the transmission of the parasitosis and eventually reduce the disease. Progress has been made in the development of vaccines for the prevention of porcine cysticercosis. In our research group, three peptides have been identified that, expressed synthetically (S3Pvac) or recombinantly (S3Pvac-phage), reduced the amount of cysticerci by 98.7% and 87%, respectively, in pigs exposed to natural conditions of infection. Considering that cysticercosis is orally acquired, it seems feasible to develop an edible vaccine, which could be administered by the pig farmers, simplifying the logistical difficulties of its application, reducing costs, and facilitating the implementation of vaccination programs. This chapter describes the most important advances towards the development of an oral vaccine against porcine cysticercosis.

Keywords: cysticercosis, *T. solium*, oral vaccine, transgenic plant, *Carica papaya*

1. Introduction

Taenia solium taeniasis/cysticercosis is a parasitic zoonosis that significantly affect economic and public health. Neurocysticercosis (NCC) is a most severe form of the disease caused by the establishment of the larval stage (cysticerci) of *Taenia solium* in the central nervous system (CNS). In 2010, the World Health Organization declared it one of the leading neglected diseases and aims to develop strategies for its eradication and prevention [1].

Between control measures it has been explored the improvement of health education, sanitary conditions, standards of meat inspection and the rearing of pigs. It has also been explored the impact of massive or individual treatment of taeniasis and the treatment and/or vaccination of pigs, all of them with promising results [2–4]. Vaccination of pigs would imply an unlikely immediate and potent effect upon the number of tapeworm-carriers in rural communities, interrupting the parasite's life cycle and eventually reduce human neurocysticercosis. Developing an effective vaccine against *T. solium* pig cysticercosis is also being pursued by different research groups with promising results [5, 6].

In our group, an anti-cysticercosis vaccine named S3Pvac based on three peptides expressed was developed. The vaccine synthetically (S3Pvac) or recombinant (S3Pvac-phage) produced, reduced the number of cysticerci by 98.7% and 87% [7, 8] in randomized field trials, respectively. The recombinant vaccine was subsequently used in a control program applied in the State of Guerrero, confirming its usefulness. Indeed, S3Pvac-phage significantly reduce the prevalence of porcine cysticercosis from 7 to 0.5% and 3.6 to 0.3% estimated by tongue examination or ultrasound, respectively [3]. In the course of this control program, we were able to evaluate the difficulties involved in using an injectable vaccine. Pigs are produced free rurally reared, thus the application of an injectable vaccine requires their capture and subjection, a laborious procedure that increases the costs of vaccination and limits its massive application. Considering that cysticercosis is orally acquired, it seems feasible to develop an oral vaccine [9], which could be administered by the pig breeder, simplifying the logistical difficulties of its administration, reducing costs and facilitating the implementation of vaccination control programs.

For the design of an oral vaccine the use of plants is increasingly recognized as valuable platform. Plants offer the production of antigens at low costs, circumventing costly purification procedures. Plants also offer a natural way of antigen encapsulation preventing its degradation by the detrimental environment to which an oral intake vaccine is exposed such us antigen degradation by low pH, mucosal enzymes [10, 11] and the use of cell cultures will avoid non-desirable environmental effects due to the release of transgenic plants into the environment.

Moreover, plants also frequently include components with adjuvant properties like saponins that may increase the immunogenicity of the vaccine [12]. Considering this, the recombinant peptides KETc7, KETc1.6His, and KETc12.6His were expressed in transgenic clones of papaya embryogenic calli [13]. The three clones together constitute the oral S3Pvac-papaya vaccine candidate. Papaya was selected because the high efficiency of transformation and its own antiparasitic properties [14].

This third version of the vaccine has been shown to be immunogenic in mice and pigs and is being produced in suspended culture systems to massively produced this oral version of the vaccine that must be evaluated on the field against pig cysticercosis.

2. Parasite and oral immunity

Oral vaccination is an interest route to prevent infections caused by orally acquired pathogens overcoming the limitations of current injection-based vaccines in providing front-line protection against pathogen invasion and dissemination [15]. It offers a painless, safe and low-cost route that does not require trained personnel. Moreover, this route can elicit mucosal and systemic immunity. Vaccine antigen can be recognized and translocated by M cells, which act as sentinels and enter directly into the Peyer's patches. Then antigens can be transported to the intestinal mesenteric lymph nodes, stimulating the host's systemic and mucosal immune response resulting in the production of IgA and IgG antibodies with the ability to neutralize of invading pathogens before they are able to cause a widespread infection. Oral vaccination can also trigger an effective cellular immunity. However, the development of oral vaccines is a major challenge due to an inefficient

Pathogen	Plant	Protein	Route	Species	Reference
Rabies virus	Tomato	GP	ND	ND	[16]
Hemorrhagic Virus	Potato	VP60	Sc, Im	Rabbit	[17]
Rotavirus A	Potato	VP6	Ip	Mice	[18]
Foot and mouth virus	Arabidopsis	VP1	Ip	Mice	[19]
Foot and mouth virus	Potato	VP1	Ip	Mice	[20]
Foot and mouth virus	Alfalfa	Peptide VP1 β-glucuronidase	Ip	Mice*	[21]
Gastroenteritis virus	Arabidopsis	GP- S	Im	Mice	[22]
Gastroenteritis virus	Potato	GP- S	Oral	Mice	[23]
Gastroenteritis virus	Tobacco	GP- S	Ip	Pig	[24]
Gastroenteritis virus	Seeds of corn	GP- S	Oral	Pig*	[25, 26]
S3Pvac-papaya	Embryogenic Transgenic clones	KETc1, KETc12 and KETc7 peptides	Sc	Mice	[13]
S3Pvac-papaya	Embryogenic Transgenic clones	KETc1, KETc12 and KETc7 peptides	Oral	Pig	[27]

**Protection against infection.*
Sc: subcutaneous; Im: intramuscular; Ip: intraperitoneal, ND: Not determined; GP: Glycoprotein.

Table 1.
Expression of antigens aimed at veterinary vaccine development.

transport to reach M cells and the possibility to induce local and systemic immune tolerance. Considering that plant-based vaccines usually expressed low content of antigen it seems feasible to avoid oral tolerance using the proper dose and vaccine schedule. It remains to be elucidated if plants-derived vaccines could overcome mucosal tolerance when administered to human beings.

Table 1 shows various plants that have been used to express antigens from different pathogens to be evaluated as edible vaccines. Tobacco has been used as an experimental model of transformation and expression. However, the use of other species such as tomatoes, lettuce, potatoes, corn, soybeans, alfalfa, Arabidopsis, papaya and carrots has been expanded [11, 28–33]. In some of these plants, the expressed recombinant antigen has shown efficacy when evaluated in experimental models or directly in the naturally affected host. Recombinant antigens have been reported to induce an immune response with the production of IgG, IgM or IgA antibodies, regardless of the route of administration [31].

3. Transgenic plant platform

Many different advantages of expression of recombinant proteins in transgenic plants for vaccine production can be mentioned over other commonly expression systems, such as bacteria, yeasts and baculoviruses. Plants can be constitutively or tissue-specific expressed in single or multiple transgenes, antigens can be stable in seeds without the requirement of refrigeration, no purification nor cold chain for preservation.

Transgenic plants can also be used as bioreactors to produce high amounts of the recombinant protein of interest [34, 35]. They can also be produced as *in vitro* tissue culture, cell suspensions, hairy roots, moss protonema, microalgae and whole plants. There are many experimental plant-made veterinary vaccines produced in seeds, fruits, and leaves, that can be orally delivered as part of the animal feed, thus offering great convenience and economy in immunizing large populations of animals on farms [35]. The expression of antigens for the production of vaccines in transgenic plants is considered a safe and effective immunization system, which can avoid some of the difficulties associated with traditional vaccination methods, as well as a reduction in the costs of production, distribution and conservation.

One nice study of veterinary interest is the expression of the glycoprotein S of the porcine gastroenteritis virus in corn seeds for the production of an oral vaccine, which has also the ability to induce protection, through colostrum, in piglets [25, 26].

3.1 *Carica papaya* L.

Classification of *Carica papaya L.*
Family: *Caricaceae.*
Gender: *Carica.*
Species: *C. papaya L.*
Morphological type: Arboreal.
Climate: Equatorial tropical.

Carica papaya is a species of pantropical plant that grow in tropical regions of the Americas from Mexico to Argentina, Africa and Asia. The main importers are: United States, Japan, Hong Kong and the European Union. *Carica papaya* is known by different common names such as capaidso, naimi, nampucha, pucha, fruit bomb, milky, mamao, pawpaw. Papaya is an arborescent, semi-perennial plant that grows in areas with an average rainfall of 1800 mm per year and an average annual temperature of 20–22°C, a large number of varieties have been developed. Papaya fruiting occurs 10 to 12 months after transplantation, is maintained for ten years, and female, male or hermaphrodite [36] trees can be obtained. Papaya is a fruit known for its nutritional benefits and medicinal properties. Main papaya components and their reported properties are shown in **Table 2**.

3.2 *Carica papaya* as a cestode vaccine

Papaya is an alternative system for the exploration of tropical tree genomes, containing a genome of 372 megabase (Mb), of diploid inheritance with 9 pairs of chromosomes and presents the smallest gene number, 24,746 genes [37]. Papaya exhibits some properties of possible advantages to be used as a platform to express *T. solium* vaccine antigens. Papaya components have antiparasitic properties per se [14]. Cells can be easily transformed by bioballistics and *in vitro* propagated and regenerated [38].

Among many papaya components, the papain contained in the latex has been widely evaluated in its ability to damage the cuticle of intestinal parasites by proteolytic digestion. **Table 3** shows some reports on the characterization and evaluation of antiparasitic activity of papaya against *Trichostrongylus colubrormis, Heligmosomoides polygyrus, Trichuris muris, Protospirura muricola* [39, 44–49] *Rodentolepis microstoma* [39], *Hymenolepis diminuta and microstoma* [40].

Composition		**Properties**	
Nutrimental	**Enzymatic**	**Fruit**	**Seed**
Carbohydrates	Papain	Digestive	Oxytocic
Sugars	Chymopapain	Healing	Vermifuge
Food fiber	Caricain	Strengthens Immunity	Spermatocide
Fat	Glycyl endopeptidase	Antibacterial	Emmenagogue
Proteins	**Lesser amounts**	Contraceptive	
Retinol (vit. A)	Class II chitinase	Analgesic	
β-carotene	Class III chitinase	Antibiotic	
Thiamine (vit. B_1)	Serin protease inhibitor	Stimulation of pancreatic juices	
Riboflavin (vit. B_2)	Glutamyl cyclotransferase	Hypotensive	
Niacin (vit. B_3)	Beta-1,3-glucanase	Febrifuge	
Pantothenic acid (vit. B_5)	Cystatin	Anti-inflammatory	
Folic acid (vit. B_9)	Acetogenins*	Anti-helminthic	
Vitamin C	Carpasemine		
Vitamin E			
Vitamin K			

**Antiparasitic activity. Calcium, iron, magnesium, manganese, phosphorus, potassium, sodium and Zn are also included in papaya.*

Table 2.
Papaya components and medicinal properties reported.

Evaluation	**Component**	**Treatment**	**Results**	**Reference**
In vitro				
Rodentolepis microstoma	Papain (Sigma) Raw latex (Sigma)	25 mM	Disrupt the surface of the cuticle	[39]
Hymenolepis diminuta microstoma	Latex supernatant Commercial papain	Not available	Damage to the strobile Reduced motility and subsequent death of the parasite	[40]
Anoplocephala perfoliata	Cysteine-proteinases Latex supernatant	300 mM	Reduced motility and induced death of the parasite	[41]
Hymenolepis diminuta	Papaya latex supernatant	2.4 μmol	Affected worm growth	[42]
In vivo **(mouse)**				
Hymenolepis microstoma	Latex supernatant	240 nm for 6 days	Minimal and temporary efficacy	[43]

Table 3.
Antiparasitic activity of papaya against some cestodes.

Anoplocephala perfoliate [41] *Hymenolepis diminuta* [42] *Hymenolepis microstoma* [43] without causing side effects to the host [50, 51].

3.3 S3Pvac-papaya anticysticercosis vaccine

For the development of the S3Pvac-papaya cysticercosis vaccine, three genetic constructions were used for the expression of recombinant peptides, KETc1.6His, KETc12.6His and KETc7 [13]. **Figure 1** summarize the methodology employed for the production of S3Pvac-papaya vaccine.

3.4 Protective properties of S3Pvac papaya against cysticercosis

The S3Pvac vaccine expressed in embryogenic papaya clones has demonstrated high protective capacity against experimental murine and *T. pisiformis* cysticercosis orally administered. **Table 4** shows the protective effect induced by oral immunization in mice at a dose range of 0.1 to 1 μg of soluble extract, whilst a higher dose lowered the percent of protection. In addition, different vaccine formulations also reduced the expected parasite load. On the other hand, the oral vaccine significantly reduced the number of infected rabbits and the percentage of cysticercus-free animals (83%), 21 days after the infection. The S3Pvac-papaya vaccine has not yet been evaluated in pigs, however, its immunogenic response in mice and pigs [27, 52], and its protective capacity in different models exhibit its potential to exert a protective response against naturally acquired porcine cysticercosis.

We previously reported non-specific protection that was induced by the wild type soluble extract [52, 54] has been attributed to the antiparasitic properties described to papaya itself mentioned above.

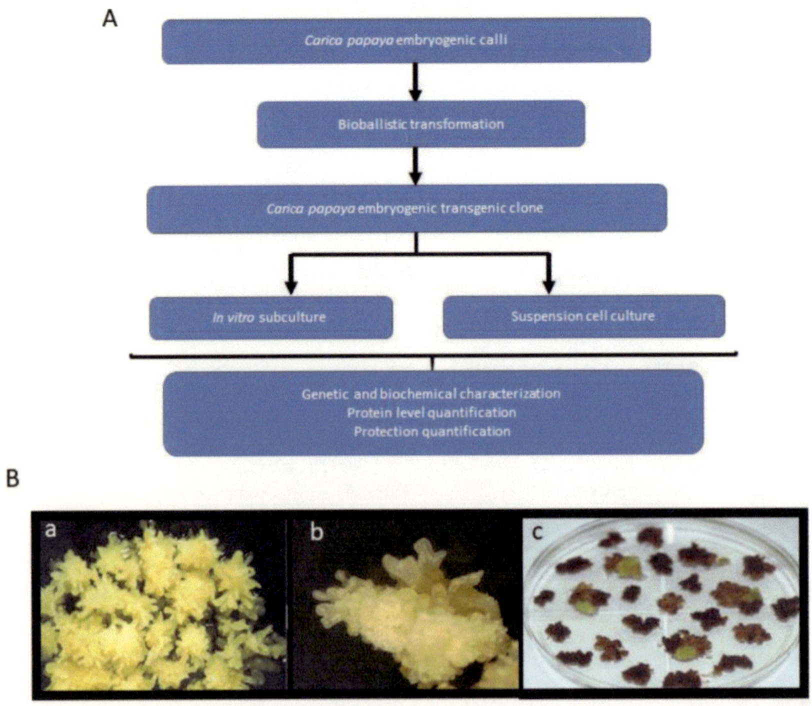

Figure 1.
(A) Production of transgenic embryogenic papaya clones by a bioballistic method (B) Embryogenic papaya callus: a) Induction of embryogenic callus; b) Embryos in globular stage for transformation; c) Selection of transformed clones in selective medium.

Experimental model	Immunized with:	Mean ± SD (% Protection)†	Immune response	Reference
				[27]
	Saline	27.2 ± 14.2		
	S3Pvac papaya saline (μg/dose)			
Murine *T. crassiceps* cysticercosis	0.1	12.3 ± 3.4* (55)	CD4, CD8 proliferation	
	1	10.8 ± 2.5* (60)	CD4, CD8 proliferation	
	10	9.2 ± 1.0* (66)	Specific IgG Abs; CD4 and CD8 proliferation	
	100	41.4 ± 62 (0)		[52]
	Saline	18.6 ± 17.3* (86.8)		
	Corn starch§	29.8 ± 31.4 (41.4)		[27]
	Soy oil	10.3 ± 2.2* (75)		
	Canola oil	11.5 ± 8.6* (84)		
Rabbit experimental *T. pisiformis*	Saline	4.33 ± 4.01		[53]
	S3Pvac papaya£	0.25 ± 0.62* (94)		

†*Mean ± standard deviation of the number of cysticerci recovered in each group.*
§*Mice were fed with S3Pvac-papaya soluble extract (1 μg of total protein) into different vehicles.*
£*Rabbits received a suspension of 20 mg of each embryogenic transgenic papaya clone expressing KETc1, KETc12 and KETc7 in a gelatin capsule.*
**Protection statistically significant (P < 0.05).*

Table 4.
Protective capacity induced by oral S3Pvac-papaya vaccine against experimental.

3.5 Biotechnological approach for the production of papaya anti-cysticercosis vaccine

Plant biotechnology is a rapidly evolving area with major impact in the production of molecules with high pharmaceutical value. *In vitro* culture techniques offer central advantages in the manufacture of desired chemicals for human health. The benefits include a systematic supply of compounds under optimized controlled conditions, independence of weather, soil, disease, and socio-political problems; discovery of new compounds, bio-transformation systems and better adaptation to market changes. In an inclusive context, *in vitro* systems will give a better understanding of plant biochemistry and physiology, as well as some basic aspects of plant differentiation.

Plant biotechnology involves relevant procedures in the manufacture of oral vaccines enabling the production of higher amounts of active biomasses from transgenic plants, by means of massive propagation of cells, tissues and organs [12, 55]. Among others, these procedures include the growth of callus (aggregates of undifferentiated cells growing in solid media), suspension cultures (individualized undifferentiated cells growing in liquid media); as well as embryo cultures that could be grown in solid or in liquid nutrient media.

The three callus lines expressing KETc1, KETc7 and KETc12 peptides were generated, and further efforts to optimize the massive growth of the corresponding callus and suspension cultures, were conducted. These *in vitro* systems constitute adequate platforms for the massive production of papaya anti-cysticercosis vaccine in the near future.

3.5.1 Callus cultures

In the establishment and optimization of callus cell lines, *Carica papaya* L. (KETc7) embryogenic calli were used to obtain friable undifferentiated cells. Calli were placed in solid culture medium with 30 g/L sucrose, 3 g/L^{-}polivinilpilorridone and 1.5 g/L^{-}of phytagel. The nutrient media MS [56] and B5 [57] were evaluated; and the presence of the phytoregulators 2,4-dichlorophenoxyacetic acid (2,4-D) at 1.0, 2.0 and 3.0 mg/L^{-}combined with kinetin (KN) at 1.0, 2.0 and 3.0 mg/L’ was also tested. The cultures were maintained at 25°C and subjected to constant light as well as dark conditions. The best results were obtained for callus growing in B5 medium with 2 mgL^{-1} of 2,4-D combined with 2 mgL^{-1} KN in dark conditions (**Figure 2**). In these conditions after two subcultures non-phenolized calluses were developed, and after several subcultures the friable callus KETc7 cell line, was established.

3.5.2 Cell suspension cultures

Ten grams fresh weight (FW) of the friable callus line KETc7 were inoculated in 250 ml Erlenmeyer baffled flasks containing 100 ml nutrient medium without phytagel, and placed for 30 days on a rotary shaker at 100 rpm, 25°C and dark conditions. To disaggregate cell clusters and increase oxygen transfer, baffled flasks were used (**Figure 3**).

The cultures were sub-cultured in fresh medium every 15 days, and the best results were observed when using B5 nutrient medium, cultivated in darkness, and producing uniform suspended cultures without phenolization (**Figure 4**).

Cell viability was maintained at 95% until 45 days in culture, as confirmed by the fluorescein diacetate (FDA) method (**Figure 5**) [58].

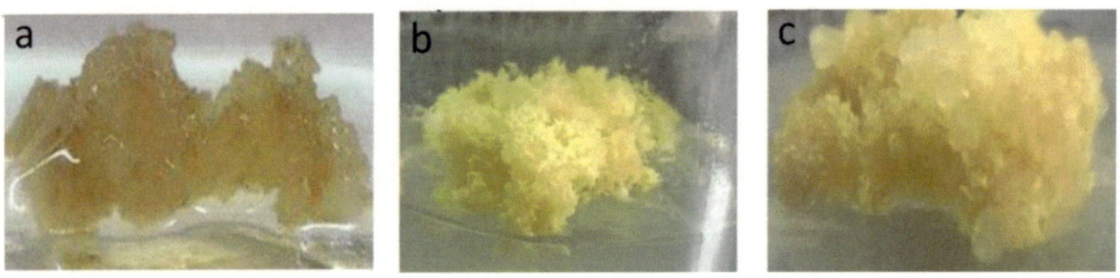

Figure 2.
Optimization of C. papaya KETc7 callus cell line under different growth conditions. (a) Photoperiod, (b) constant light, (c) darkness.

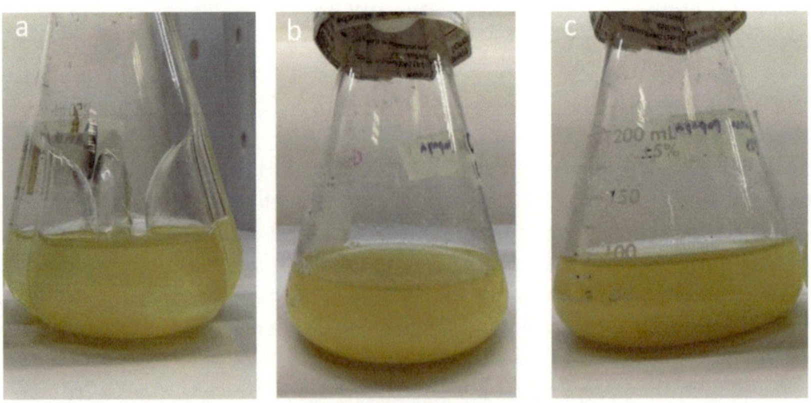

Figure 3.
Establishment of C. papaya KETc7 cell suspension line. (a) Culture in baffle flasks at 15 days (b) culture in Erlenmeyer flasks at 15 days (c) culture in Erlenmeyer flasks at 30 days.

Once the friable uniform cell suspension cell line was established, it became possible to evaluate the growth kinetics of the culture during 45 days by collecting samples every 3 days, and determining the following growth parameters: fresh weight, dry weight, cell viability, pH and carbohydrate consumption [59].

The results showed that the KETc7 suspension cell line grew very well, reaching a doubling time of 6.9 days and a specific growth rate (μ) of 0.10 d^{-1}. The maximum biomass value was 14.36 gPS L^{-1} obtained at 15 days in culture.

3.5.3 Embryo suspension cultures

The KETc7 embryos callus cell line generated in solid B5 medium without phytoregulators was used to establish embryo suspension cultures. An inoculum of 10% was added into 250 ml Erlenmeyer flasks containing 100 ml of liquid B5 medium (**Figure 6**). The flasks were kept on an orbital shaker at a stirring speed of 115 rpm, under constant light conditions (24 $\mu mol.m^{-2}$. S^{-1}) and 25°C. After 15 days, the biomass was sub cultivated in the same conditions described above, and the culture was propagated.

3.5.4 Cell suspension cultures in bioreactors

To scale-up the *C. papaya* suspension cultures 2 L airlift bioreactors were employed, with the following geometric design: height (52 cm), diameter (7 cm), draft tube height (27 cm), diameter of inner draft tube (2.7 cm), and bottom clearance (2.0 cm) [60]. The air was sprayed at the bottom of the draft, generating an internal loop in which the upcomer is in the draft, and the downcomer in the ring.

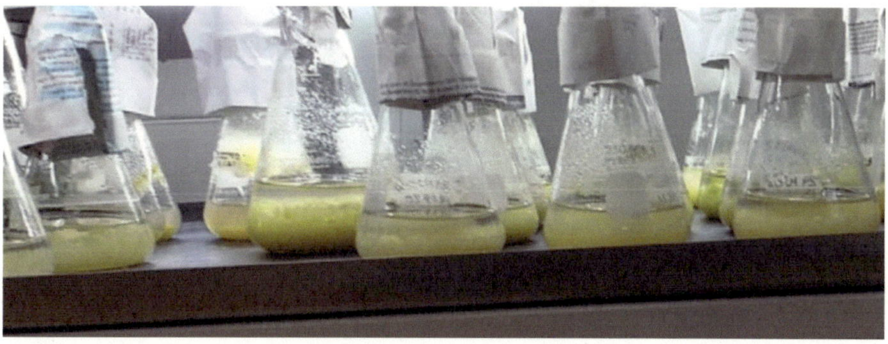

Figure 4.
Growth of C. papaya KETc7 cell suspension line at 15 days in a rotary shaker at 100 rpm, 25°C, in the dark.

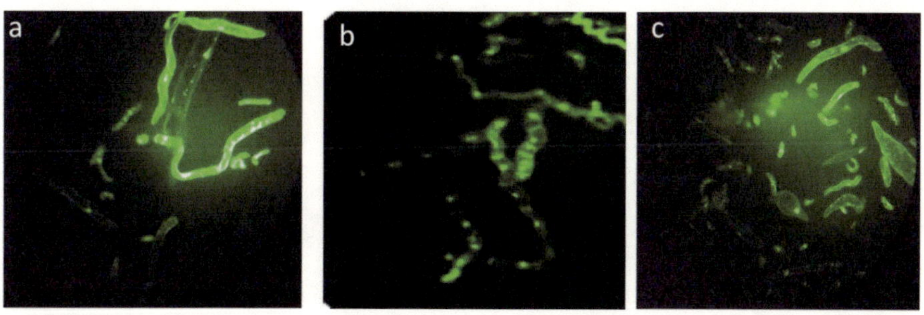

Figure 5.
Cell viability of C. papaya KETc7 cell suspension line by the fluorescein diacetate (FDA) method at day a) 0, b) 7, and c) 15, in an Epifluorescence Microscope Nikon Eclipse E400 (40X).

The bioreactor was sterilized and then filled with autoclaved B5 medium (1.8 L) supplemented with 30 g/L sucrose, 2,4-D and KN (2 mg/L each). Fifteen-days-old *C. papaya* KETc7 cell suspension line was used to obtain an inoculum of 10% (v/v) FW. The culture in bioreactor was incubated at 25 ± 2°C under continuous light (white light flux density of 50 μmol/m^2/s) for 30 days. The bioreactor was operated in a batch mode at 0.1 vvm for 15 days and subsequently at 0.8 vvm, until the end of the culture period. Under these conditions, an adequate mixing of the cell suspension was obtained. Antifoam (Dow Corning FG-10) was applied as required, by injection of 0.5 mL (0.1% v/v). The culture was sampled every three days and the concentration of biomass, pH and sugars, was determined. Results show that the K ETc7 cell suspension culture was able to grow uniformly and that the exponential growth phase was reached from days 6 to 12, followed by a stationary phase. The maximum biomass was of 18.6 ± 0.7 g/L DW (**Figure** 7).

3.5.5 Embryo suspension cultures in bioreactors

Growth of *C. papaya* KETc7 embryo suspension line was scaled-up in the 2 L airlift bioreactors described before. Two weeks old embryo suspension line was used to obtain an inoculum of 10% (v/v) FW. The culture in bioreactor was incubated at 25 ± 2°C under continuous light (white light flux density of 50 μmol/m^2/s)

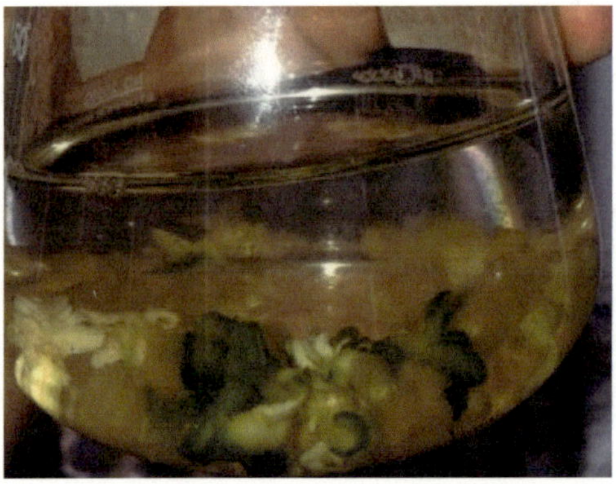

Figure 6.
C. papaya KETc7 embryo suspension line grown in B5 medium at 100 rpm, 25°C, and constant light (24 μmol. m^{-2}. S^{-1}).

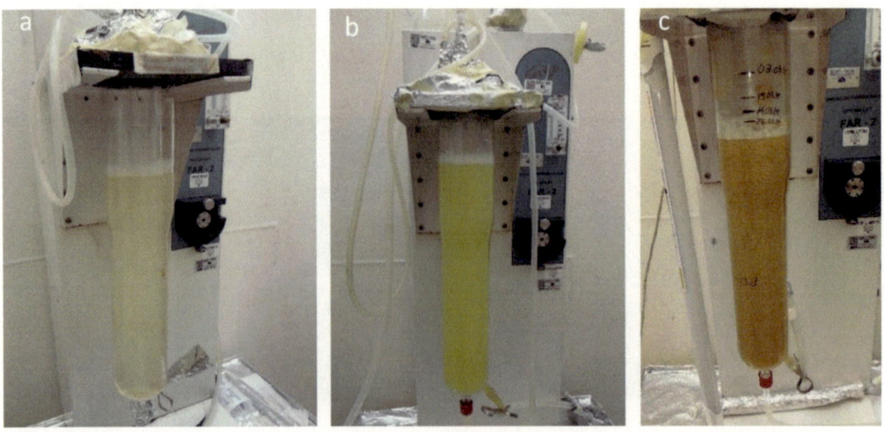

Figure 7.
C. papaya KETc7 cell suspension line growing in airlift bioreactor: (a) day 0, (b) day 15, (c) day 30.

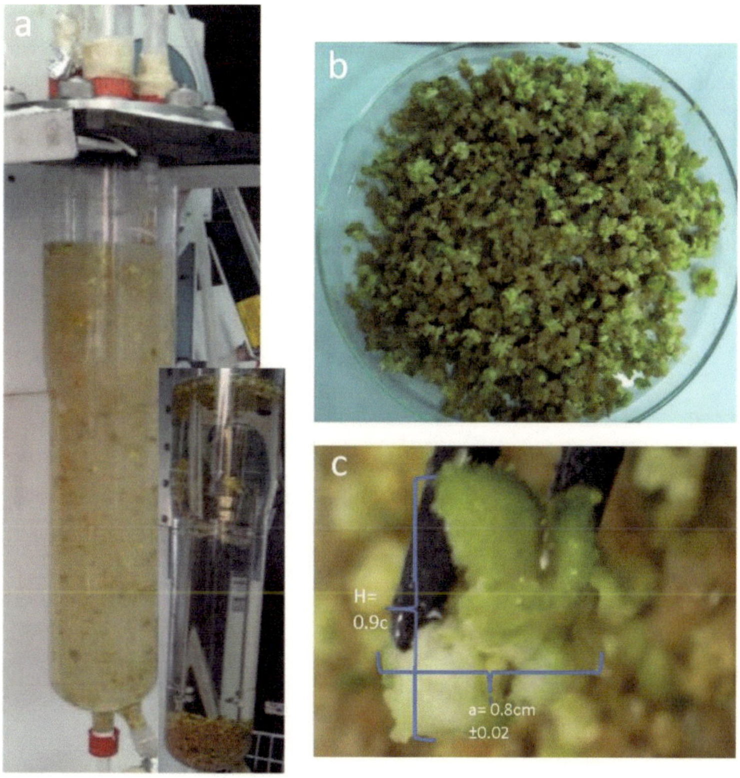

Figure 8.
C. papaya KETc7 embryo suspension line growing in airlift bioreactor (a) embryo culture in airlift bioreactor at 30 days, (b) harvested embryos after 30 days in culture, (c) embryos observed in stereoscopic microscope (10×).

for 30 days. The bioreactor was operated in a batch mode at 0.1 vvm for 15 days and subsequently at 0.8 vvm until the end of the culture period. Embryo culture of the line KETc7in bioreactor batch type process, showed uniform growth. A maximum biomass of 30 g/L DW was obtained, which represents 4 times more respect to the initial inoculum and the number of generated embryos was of 279 (**Figure 8**).

4. Conclusions

This review addresses oral vaccination as a feasible approach to prevent parasitic diseases. Since most anti-parasitic vaccines currently available are parenterally administered, their use involves high production and logistic costs and become inaccessible for underdeveloped countries. To cope with this issue, the use of papaya transgenic clones is herein proposed to develop an anti-cysticercosis oral vaccine and to assay its effectiveness against other parasitic infections of veterinary and/or public health interest. The use of biotechnological tools by escalation of suspension cultures would allow us to produce a vaccine in sufficient, controlled amounts for its direct application, reducing the use of antibiotics, and therefore the risk of bacterial resistance.

Acknowledgements

Thanks to Georgina Díaz, B.Sc., and Gonzalo Acero, B.Sc., for their technical support. Special thanks to Juan Francisco Rodríguez, B.Sc., for his help in preparing the original manuscript. This work was supported by the Programa de Investigación para el Desarrollo y la Optimización de Vacunas, Inmunomoduladores y Métodos Diagnósticos, Institute of Biomedical Research, UNAM.

Conflict of interest

The authors declare no conflict of interest.

Author details

Marisela Hernández[1†], Anabel Ortiz Caltempa[2†], Jacquelynne Cervantes[1], Nelly Villalobos[3], Cynthia Guzmán[2], Gladis Fragoso[1], Edda Sciutto[1*] and María Luisa Villareal[2]

1 Institute of Biomedical Research, National Autonomous University of Mexico, School Circuit, University City, Mexico City, Mexico

2 Biotechnology Research Center, Autonomous University of the State of Morelos, Cuernavaca, Mexico

3 Faculty of Veterinary Medicine and Zootechnics, National Autonomous University of Mexico, School Circuit, University City, Mexico City, Mexico

*Address all correspondence to: edda@unam.mx

† These authors contributed equally.

References

[1] WHO. The Control of Neglected Zoonotic Diseases-Report of the third conference organized with ICONZ, DFID-RIU, Gates Foundation, SOS, EU, TDR and FAO with the participation of ILRI and OIE WHO headquarters, Geneva, Switzerland 23-24 november 2010. 2010.

[2] Gabriël S, Dorny P, Mwape KE, Trevisan C, Braae UC, Magnussen P *et al.* Control of Taenia solium taeniasis/cysticercosis: The best way forward for sub-Saharan Africa? Acta Trop 2017; **165:** 252-260.

[3] De Aluja AS, Suárez-Marín R, Sciutto-Conde E, Morales-Soto J, Martínez-Maya JJ, Villalobos N. Evaluación del impacto de un programa de control de la teniasis-cisticercosis (*Taenia solium)* [Evaluation of the impact of a control program against taeniasis-cysticercosis (Taenia solium)]. Salud Publica Mex 2014; **56**: 259.

[4] Garcia HH, Gonzalez AE, Tsang VCW, O'Neal SE, Llanos-Zavalaga F, Gonzalvez G *et al.* Elimination of Taenia solium Transmission in Northern Peru. N Engl J Med 2016; **374**: 2335-2344.

[5] Gauci C, Jayashi C, Lightowlers MW. Vaccine development against the taenia solium parasite: The role of recombinant protein expression in Escherichia coli. Bioengineered 2013; **4**. doi:10.4161/bioe.23003.

[6] Sciutto E, Fragoso G, Hernández M, Rosas G, Martínez JJ, Fleury A *et al.* Development of the S3Pvac vaccine against murine taenia crassiceps cysticercosis: A historical review. J Parasitol 2013; **99**: 693-702.

[7] Huerta M, De Aluja AS, Fragoso G, Toledo A, Villalobos N, Hernández M *et al.* Synthetic peptide vaccine against Taenia solium pig cysticercosis: Successful vaccination in a controlled field trial in rural Mexico. Vaccine 2001; **20**: 262-266.

[8] Morales J, Martínez JJ, Manoutcharian K, Hernández M, Fleury A, Gevorkian G *et al.* Inexpensive anti-cysticercosis vaccine: S3Pvac expressed in heat inactivated M13 filamentous phage proves effective against naturally acquired Taenia solium porcine cysticercosis. Vaccine 2008; **26**: 2899-2905.

[9] Cripps AW, Kyd JM, Foxwell AR. Vaccines and mucosal immunisation. In: *Vaccine*. Vaccine, 2001, pp. 2513-2515.

[10] Mason G, Provero P, Vaira AM, Accotto GP. Estimating the number of integrations in transformed plants by quantitative real-time PCR. BMC Biotechnol 2002; **2**. doi:10.1186/1472-6750-2-20.

[11] Walmsley AM, Arntzen CJ. Plants for delivery of edible vaccines. Curr Opin Biotechnol 2000; **11**: 126-129.

[12] Rosales-Mendoza S, Salazar-González JA. Immunological aspects of using plant cells as delivery vehicles for oral vaccines. Expert Rev Vaccines 2014; **13**: 737-749.

[13] Hernández M, Cabrera-Ponce JL, Fragoso G, López-Casillas F, Guevara-García A, Rosas G *et al.* A new highly effective anticysticercosis vaccine expressed in transgenic papaya. Vaccine 2007; **25**: 4252-4260.

[14] Stepek G, Behnke JM, Buttle DJ, Duce IR. Natural plant cysteine proteinases as anthelmintics? Trends Parasitol 2004; **20**: 322-327.

[15] Miquel-Clopés A, Bentley EG, Stewart JP, Carding SR. Mucosal vaccines and technology. Clin Exp Immunol 2019; **196**: 205-214.

[16] McGarvey PB, Hammond J, Dienelt MM, Hooper DC, Fang Fu Z, Dietzschold B *et al.* Expression of the rabies virus glycoprotein in transgenic tomatoes. Bio/Technology 1995; **13**: 1484-1487.

[17] Castañón S, Marín MS, Martín-Alonso JM, Boga JA, Casais R, Humara JM *et al.* Immunization with Potato Plants Expressing VP60 Protein Protects against Rabbit Hemorrhagic Disease Virus. J Virol 1999; **73**: 4452-4455.

[18] Matsumura T, Itchoda N, Tsunemitsu H. Production of immunogenic VP6 protein of bovine group A rotavirus in transgenic potato plants: Brief report. Arch Virol 2002; **147**: 1263-1270.

[19] Carrillo C, Wigdorovitz A, Oliveros JC, Zamorano PI, Sadir AM, Gómez N *et al.* Protective Immune Response to Foot-and-Mouth Disease Virus with VP1 Expressed in Transgenic Plants. J Virol 1998; **72**: 1688-1690.

[20] Carrillo C, Wigdorovitz A, Trono K, Dus Santos MJ, Castañón S, Sadir AM *et al.* Induction of a virus-specific antibody response to foot and mouth disease virus using the structural protein VP1 expressed in transgenic potato plants. Viral Immunol 2001; **14**: 49-57.

[21] Dus Santos MJ, Wigdorovitz A, Trono K, Ríos RD, Franzone PM, Gil F *et al.* A novel methodology to develop a foot and mouth disease virus (FMDV) peptide-based vaccine in transgenic plants. Vaccine 2002; **20**: 1141-1147.

[22] Gómez N, Carrillo C, Salinas J, Parra F, Borca M V., Escribano JM. Expression of immunogenic glycoprotein S polypeptides from transmissible gastroenteritis coronavirus in transgenic plants. Virology 1998; **249**: 352-358.

[23] Gómez N, Wigdorovitz A, Castañón S, Gil F, Ordá R, Borca M V. *et al.* Oral immunogenicity of the plant derived spike protein from swine-transmissible gastroenteritis coronavirus. Arch Virol 2000; **145**: 1725-1732.

[24] Tuboly T, Yu W, Bailey A, Degrandis S, Du S, Erickson L *et al.* Immunogenicity of porcine transmissible gastroenteritis virus spike protein expressed in plants. Vaccine 2000; **18**: 2023-2028.

[25] Streatfield SJ, Jilka JM, Hood EE, Turner DD, Bailey MR, Mayor JM *et al.* Plant-based vaccines: Unique advantages. Vaccine 2001; **19**: 2742-2748.

[26] Lamphear BJ, Streatfield SJ, Jilka JM, Brooks CA, Barker DK, Turner DD *et al.* Delivery of subunit vaccines in maize seed. J Control Release 2002; **85**: 169-180.

[27] Fragoso G, Hernández M, Cervantes-Torres J, Ramírez-Aquino R, Chapula H, Villalobos N *et al.* Transgenic papaya: a useful platform for oral vaccines. Planta 2017; **245**: 1037-1048.

[28] Floss DM, Falkenburg D, Conrad U. Production of vaccines and therapeutic antibodies for veterinary applications in transgenic plants: An overview. Transgenic Res 2007; **16**: 315-332.

[29] Rosales-Mendoza S, Soria-Guerra RE, López-Revilla R, Moreno-Fierros L, Alpuche-Solís ÁG. Ingestion of transgenic carrots expressing the Escherichia coli heat-labile enterotoxin B subunit protects mice against cholera toxin challenge. Plant Cell Rep 2008; **27**: 79-84.

[30] Sala F, Rigano MM, Barbante A, Basso B, Walmsley AM, Castiglione S. Vaccine antigen production in transgenic plants: Strategies, gene constructs and perspectives. In: *Vaccine*. Vaccine, 2003, pp. 803-808.

[31] Streatfield SJ, Howard JA. Plant-based vaccines. Int J Parasitol 2003; **33**: 479-493.

[32] Streatfield SJ. Mucosal immunization using recombinant plant-based oral vaccines. Methods 2006; **38**: 150-157.

[33] Tacket CO. Plant-derived vaccines against diarrheal diseases. Vaccine 2005; **23**:1866-1869.

[34] Xu J, Towler M, Weathers PJ. Platforms for Plant-Based Protein Production. 2018 doi:10.1007/978-3-319-54600-1_14.

[35] Massa S, Presenti O, Benvenuto E. Engineering Plants for the Future: Farming with Value-Added Harvest. Springer, Cham, 2018, pp. 65-108.

[36] Agricultura. El cultivo de la papaya. https://www.infoagro.com/frutas/frutas_tropicales/papaya.htm [Accessed: 19 February 2021].

[37] Ming R, Hou S, Feng Y, Yu Q, Dionne-Laporte A, Saw JH *et al.* The draft genome of the transgenic tropical fruit tree papaya (Carica papaya Linnaeus). Nature 2008; **452**: 991-996.

[38] Cabrera-Ponce JL, Vegas-Garcia A, Herrera-Estrella L. Herbicide resistant transgenic papaya plants produced by an efficient particle bombardment transformation method. Plant Cell Rep 1995; **15**: 1-7.

[39] Stepek G, Curtis RHC, Kerry BR, Shewry PR, Clark SJ, Lowe AE *et al.* Nematicidal effects of cysteine proteinases against sedentary plant parasitic nematodes. Parasitology 2007; **134**: 1831-1838.

[40] Mansur F, Luoga W, Buttle DJ, Duce IR, Lowe A, Behnke JM. The anthelmintic efficacy of natural plant cysteine proteinases against two rodent cestodes Hymenolepis diminuta and Hymenolepis microstoma in vitro. Vet Parasitol 2014; **201**: 48-58.

[41] Mansur F, Luoga W, Buttle DJ, Duce IR, Lowe A, Behnke JM. The anthelmintic efficacy of natural plant cysteine proteinases against the rat tapeworm Hymenolepis diminuta in vivo. J Helminthol 2016; **90**: 284-293.

[42] Mansur F, Luoga W, Buttle DJ, Duce IR, Lowe AE, Behnke JM. The anthelmintic efficacy of natural plant cysteine proteinases against the equine tapeworm, Anoplocephala perfoliata in vitro. J Helminthol 2016; **90**: 561-568.

[43] Mansur F, Luoga W, Buttle DJ, Duce IR, Lowe A, Behnke JM. The anthelmintic efficacy of natural plant cysteine proteinases against Hymenolepis microstoma in vivo. J Helminthol 2014; **760**: 601-611.

[44] Berger J, Asenjo CF. Anthelmintic activity of crystalline papain. *Science (80-)* 1940; **91**: 387-388.

[45] Stepek G, Lowe AE, Buttle DJ, Duce IR, Behnke JM. In vitro and in vivo anthelmintic efficacy of plant cysteine proteinases against the rodent gastrointestinal nematode, Trichuris muris. Parasitology 2006; **132**: 681-689.

[46] Stepek G, Buttle DJ, Duce IR, Behnke JM. Human gastrointestinal nematode infections: Are new control methods required? Int J Exp Pathol 2006; **87**: 325-341.

[47] Stepek G, Lowe AE, Buttle DJ, Duce IR, Behnke JM. In vitro anthelmintic effects of cysteine proteinases from plants against intestinal helminths of rodents. J Helminthol 2007; **81**: 353-360.

[48] Stepek G, Lowe AE, Buttle DJ, Duce IR, Behnke JM. The anthelmintic efficacy of plant-derived cysteine

proteinases against the rodent gastrointestinal nematode, Heligmosomoides polygyrus, in vivo. Parasitology 2007; **134**: 1409-1419.

[49] Stepek G, Lowe AE, Buttle DJ, Duce IR, Behnke JM. Anthelmintic action of plant cysteine proteinases against the rodent stomach nematode, Protospirura muricola, in vitro and in vivo. Parasitology 2007; **134**: 103-112.

[50] Hounzangbe-Adote S, Fouraste I, Moutairou K, Hoste H. In vitro effects of four tropical plants on the activity and development of the parasitic nematode, Trichostrongylus colubriformis. J Helminthol 2005; **79**: 29-33.

[51] Okeniyi JAO, Ogunlesi TA, Oyelami OA, Adeyemi LA. Effectiveness of dried Carica papaya seeds against human intestinal parasitosis: A pilot study. J Med Food 2007; **10**: 194-196.

[52] Sciutto E, Hernández M, Díaz-Orea A, Cervantes J, Rosas-Salgado G, Morales J *et al.* Towards a practical and affordable oral papaya-based vaccine: A crucial tool for taeniasis cysticercosis control programs. In: Liong M-T (ed). *Bioprocess Sciences and Technology*. Nova Science Publishers, Inc., 2011, pp. 323-338.

[53] Betancourt MA, De Aluja AS, Sciutto E, Hernández M, Bobes RJ, Rosas G *et al.* Effective protection induced by three different versions of the porcine S3Pvac anticysticercosis vaccine against rabbit experimental Taenia pisiformis cysticercosis. Vaccine 2012; **30**: 2760-2767.

[54] Hernández M, Jacquelynne G, Torres C, Luisa M, Gladis V, González F *et al.* Development of an Oral Anti-Cysticercosis Vaccine Delivered in Genetically Modified Embryogenic Callus of Papaya. *Transgenic Plant J 4* 2010.

[55] Chan HT, Daniell H. Plant-made oral vaccines against human infectious diseases-Are we there yet? Plant Biotechnol J 2015; **13**: 1056-1070.

[56] Murashige T, Skoog F. A Revised Medium for Rapid Growth and Bio Assays with Tobacco Tissue Cultures. Physiol Plant 1962; **15**: 473-497.

[57] Gamborg OL, Miller RA, Ojima K. Nutrient requirements of suspension cultures of soybean root cells. Exp Cell Res 1968; **50**: 151-158.

[58] Widholm JM. The use of fluorescein diacetate and phenosafranine for determining viability of cultured plant cells. Biotech Histochem 1972; **47**: 189-194.

[59] Pérez A. *Establecimiento de células en suspensión de C. papaya que expresan el péptido KETc7 como propuesta de una vacuna contra la cysticercosis y la hemoncosis*. Maestría en Biotecnología: Universidad Autónoma del Estado de Morelos. 2019.

[60] Caspeta L, Nieto I, Zamilpa A, Alvarez L, Quintero R, Villarreal ML. Solanum chrysotrichum hairy root cultures: Characterization, scale-up and production of five antifungal saponins for human use. Planta Med 2005; **71**: 1084-1087.

Chapter 3

Regulation of the Immune Response in Cysticercosis: Lessons from an Old Acquainted Infection

Jonadab E. Olguín and Luis Ignacio Terrazas

Abstract

In the last decades, we have learned some critical lessons about the relationship between the human body and its interaction with many infectious diseases, where regularly, the immune system has a major role in protection. We learned to differentiate between the immune response occurring in either an intracellular or extracellular parasitic infection, between innate and adaptive immune response, between either inflammatory or anti-inflammatory responses, and finally, we learned to recognize very particular mechanisms, such as the inability of the immune system to respond during very particular scenarios, such as the inability of T cells to both proliferate and produce cytokines even after their exposure to mitogens or specific-antigens. Along with our increase in the knowledge in immunology, we figured out that immunoregulation and immunosuppression are processes used by many parasites to reduce the capacity of the immune system to eliminate them, and to persist in the host favoring their transmission and also to complete their life cycles. Immunoregulation involves several mechanisms such as anergy, apoptosis, induction of both suppressive cytokines and membrane-bound molecules, as well as specialized cell populations of the immune system like regulatory T cells, Alternative Activated Macrophages, or Myeloid-derived Suppressor Cells, that together modify the outcome of the immune response. In this chapter we will review the general differences between the different types of immunoregulation, the kind of cellular populations of the immune system used by the helminths *Taenia solium* and *Taenia crassiceps* to induce immunoregulation and immunosuppression and also, the mechanisms used by these parasites such as mimicking molecules of the immune system to replace directly these mechanisms. Understanding and deciphering all these regulatory mechanisms could be useful to develop new tools to control this infection.

Keywords: Cysticercosis, Immunoregulation, Immunosuppression, *Taenia solium*, *Taenia crassiceps*, Regulatory T cells (Treg cells), Alternative Activated Macrophages (AAM), Myeloid-derived Suppressor Cells (MDSC)

1. Introduction

Taeniasis and cysticercosis, both neglected diseases, are two kinds of infections caused by the same parasite, *Taenia solium*. Taeniasis is the intestinal infection caused by the adult form of the tapeworm *T. solium*, while cysticercosis is the tissue infection caused by the larval stage, cyst or cysticercus of *T. solium* [1]. Whereas taeniasis only affects the human and it is restricted to the small intestine, cysticercosis affect two hosts, the human and the swine, besides this stage of the parasite can allocate at different anatomical sites including the brain, causing neurocysticercosis (NCC). The vast majority of medical findings by natural infection has been made during cysticercosis, given its clinical relevance when the parasite encroaches on the central nervous system including the brain and the eye [2]. In the past, NCC represented a major health problem mainly in developing countries [3], being highly prevalent in the general registration of autopsies [3]. The only way to find samples for the study of NCC, were in patients diagnosed by neuroimaging: magnetic resonance and computed tomography, and also by determination of specific antigens by ELISA and western blot from blood and cerebrospinal fluid samples [4, 5].

Because taeniasis remains asymptomatic, there are no symptoms directly associated with the disease, only general symptoms like abdominal bloating and abdominal pain [1, 5]. For this reason, a model to understand the immunological interactions between the host and the parasite and also, to understand the evolutionary capacity of *Taenia* to survive in the host was necessary. Animal models like hamsters, gerbils and chinchillas, were developed in the past to have a better understanding of the immunology in this field [6], but a limited information about it was published, having a focus in the inflammatory response in the intestinal mucosa of chinchillas receiving an immunosuppressant treatment with methyl-prednisolone [7]. Because of the nature to develop taeniasis and the necessity to have a better understanding of the immune response against *T. solium*, it was necessary to know the immunology and the mechanism of protection used by a "close familiar" to this parasite: *Taenia crassiceps*.

2. General aspects of the immune response during NCC and Taeniasis

T. crassiceps is a tapeworm that generates natural infections in some definitive canine hosts like dogs, red foxes, and wolves in the northern hemisphere of the world. It also has an extensive reproduction rate in the pleural and peritoneal cavities of their intermediate host like wild rodents [8]. For a better understanding of their life cycle, go to the reference [8]. *T. crassiceps* ORF strain was obtained by Dr. Reino Freeman in 1952. This strain has a deficient capacity to develop the scolex, therefore, cannot colonize the intestines of its definitive hosts [9]. Most of the research about the immunology of *T. crassiceps* has been developed with the ORF strain, injecting either 10 or 20 metacestodes of this parasite in the peritoneal cavity of syngenic female BALB/c mice [10, 11].

The immune response against *T. crassiceps* has been investigated in an extensive way. During the acute infection by this helminth a strong Th1 immune response characterized by high levels of IL-2 and IFN-γ is induced and has been associated with host protection, but as the infection becomes chronic, levels of both IL-2 and IFN-γ decrease as well as IL-12 produced by macrophages [12]. These reduced levels of Th1-type cytokines correlate with increased levels of IL-4 at chronic infection stages, suggesting a switch between inflammatory response in the acute infection to an anti-inflammatory response in chronic infection, favoring the adequate microenvironment for both, parasite development and their persistence in the host (**Figure 1**). Susceptibility to *T. crassiceps* infection is STAT6-mediated, characterized by strong IgG1, IgE, IL-4 and IL-13 production [13]. Therefore, unlike the case of the vast majority of helminth parasitic infections, protection during experimental cysticercosis is mediated by Th1-type immune responses, while parasite

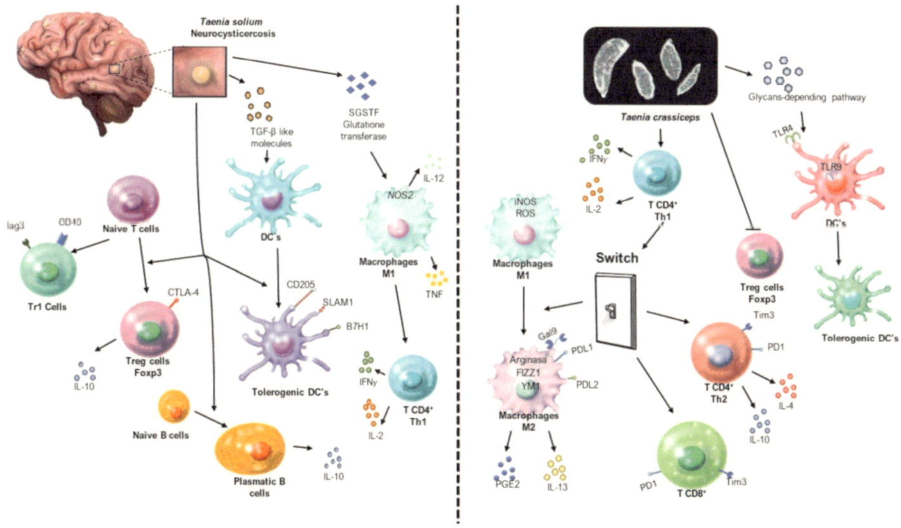

Figure 1.
Hypothetical/integrative model of immune regulation triggered by T. solium *and* T. crassiceps *infection and their released products on different types of cells. Products of both parasites can be recognized by innate cells through several pattern recognition receptors, including TLRs, CD205, among others, and induce tolerogenic DCs or modulate the activation of macrophages by inducing the expression of different inhibitory molecules in its membrane such as PDL1, PDL2, Galectin-9 (Gal-9) as well as soluble inhibitory factors such as PGE2, and IL-13, while favors the expression of genes associated with M2 polarization, such as arginase, FIZZ1 and YM1, leading to the inhibition of T cell proliferation. In contrast, the inflammatory properties of both DCs and macrophages are inhibited by these parasite molecules and the production of TNF-α, IL-12, iNOS and ROS are dramatically reduced. Additionally, TsES and TcES inhibit T cell responses through the induction of T regulatory cells as well as B regulatory cells which both are an important source of IL-10. These infections together with their secreted products can also induce a Th2-biased response and a reduced CD8 response.*

establishment is associated with Th2-type mediated immune responses [14]. One of the most relevant findings observed during experimental cysticercosis, was the reduced proliferative capacity of T lymphocytes obtained from infected mice to either nonspecific or specific antigens during chronic infection, suggesting the strong immunosuppressive capacity of *T. crassiceps* [12, 15].

On the other hand, evidence from subcutaneous, visceral, muscle, lung and cardiac tissue infected with *T. solium* in patients suggest that, out of the nervous central system (NCS), this infection causes no symptoms, reducing the possibility to understand and describe the occurring steps during early immune responses [1, 16]. Once inside of NCS, *T. solium* induces different levels of damage depending on the developing site. If the cysticercus is located in the brain parenchyma, it survives during different periods of time, from months to years, but eventually evolves in resolution [1, 2]. However, if the infection is located outside of the parenchyma's (subarachnoid) brain, it is associated with edema, inflammation and increased mortality rates around 20% in patients without a correct treatment [2, 17]. Besides its location on the NCS, also exists a relationship between the intensity of the symptomatology and the number and size of the larvae causing the infection. In fact, it was recently hypothesized that the gut-brain-axis has a major role in the manifestation of symptoms during NCC, mainly in patients with mental illness, depression and epilepsy [18], highlighting the importance for the microbiota in this field. Also, it was suggested that these interactions for the gut-brain-axis are dependent on galectin-7 (Gal-7) expression in brain endothelial cells during human *T. solium* cysticercosis [19]. Thus, the main actors for the development of cysticercosis are the host immune response, the microenvironment for the parasite development either the gut or NCS, the microbiota, and the host health status.

The immune response described in the *T. solium* rodent model has been helpful and relevant to understand the immunobiology during taeniasis and cysticercosis, being a main feature the suppression of the immune response. Next, we will try to describe both the immunoregulatory mechanisms and the direct effects of molecules secreted by *Taenia* parasites to induce immunoregulation.

3. Immunoregulation during cysticercosis

An inflammatory response during the initial infection process is necessary to induce immunity, to reduce parasite load and finally to have protection in cysticercosis. However, since basic science started to clarify the role of the immune response during cysticercosis, some special discoveries have been observed only in this helminth infection, suggesting a process of transformation from inflammation to an anti-inflammatory response, tipping the balance towards the parasite survival. Is necessary to pay attention in the fact that, during some helminth infections, the Th1 to Th2 switch is caused to keep the balance between immunity in the host with tissue repairing, and for the survival of the parasite o for its expulsion from the host, example of that are *Schistosoma mansoni*, *Nippostrongylus brasiliensis and Heligmosomoides polygyrus* infections [20, 21]. However, this Th1 to Th2 switching in cysticercosis appears to absolutely favor parasite survival. Also, this switch process is an initial step to induce an immunosuppressive process orchestrated by the parasite, or also, as a possibility, the microenvironment caused by the infection has a strong effect culminating in the incapacity to the immune response to react against the infection (**Figure 1**). Some evidence suggests that immunosuppression may be caused by T-cells, myeloid-derived cells or directly by parasite molecules like *Taenia crassiceps* excreted/secreted antigens (TcES) or *Taenia solium* excreted/secreted antigens (TsES). Also, it was suggested that asymptomatic NCC is caused by a strong period of immunosuppression by live *T. solium* parasites, because brain inflammation is not observed during the development of the infection and while the parasite remains alive [22].

3.1 Immunoregulation mediated by T-cells

During some intracellular parasitic infections, like toxoplasmosis, trypanosomiasis and leishmaniasis, an incapacity of T lymphocytes to proliferate in response to antigen-specific or polyclonal mitogens has been described, mainly during acute infection [23–26]. Although the general observation is that the process of immunosuppression starts at the beginning of the chronic *T. crassiceps* infection, it was shown that during acute intraperitoneal (ip) infection in mice, there is a significant decreased percentage of T-CD4$^+$, T-CD8$^+$ cells and B-CD19$^+$ cells at the infection site, starting at 3 days post infection (dpi) and culminating at 16 dpi [27]. These results correlate with increased levels of apoptosis, mainly in eosinophils. Perhaps, *T. crassiceps* begins to develop its suppressive microenvironment since the beginning of the development of the infection, such as reported for protozoan infections. During *T. crassiceps* chronic infection, a reduced proliferative capacity of T cells was described [12], especially in CD8-cytotoxic T cells [28]. Recent observations by our laboratory described that, this reduced capacity to induce cytotoxicity by CD8$^+$ cells is caused by increased expression of Tim-3 and PD1 molecules in an IL4-Rα, STAT-1 and IFN-γ independent-pathway (**Figure 1**, Olguin JE et al., unpublished data). Interestingly, both expression of Tim-3 and PD1 is increased in adaptive regulatory CD4$^+$Foxp3$^-$ T cells but not in natural Treg cells. In fact, during the chronic phase of experimental cysticercosis, we observed reduced percentages of Treg cells, which is contrasting with some published data. For example, a study reports that cocultured cysticerci of *T. solium* with human monocyte-derived DCs, induces Foxp3 expression in CD4$^+$ naïve T cells *in vitro* and also, increased percentage of suppressive-related molecules (**Figure 1**) [29]. The same research group showed a descriptive study in patients with NCC, observing an increased expression of natural and adaptive Treg cells in blood [30], but the authors did not show, whether these induced and natural Treg cells had the capacity to suppress another population of immune cells, for example either T-CD8 or activated CD4 T cells. Maybe, the differences observed between NCC and experimental cysticercosis in Treg cells are explained by the site where the sample was obtained (NCS and blood in *T. solium*, peritoneum in *T. crassiceps*), and by the nature of the infection. However, it is clear that, whatever scenario is observed, T cell-mediated regulation is a critical mechanism involved during the development of experimental or natural cysticercosis. Also, observations made by our group in *T. crassiceps* infection are different to those done in other helminth infections. A recent study of hookworms like *Ancylostoma duodenale*, *Necator americanus*, *Ascaris lumbricoides* and others, showed by mass cytometry a clear profile of Th2 cells, favoring increased expression of CTLA-4 in Treg cells, and B cells producing IL-10 in infected Europeans and Indonesians patients [31]. Maybe, it is necessary to describe more specific surface markers to define the population of suppressive and/or regulatory T cells. For example, it has been described as a highly suppressive T regulatory Type 1 population (Tr1) during a helminth scenario by the co-expression of CD49 and LAG-3 [32]. Tr1 cells are different from natural regulatory (Treg) cells because they do not express constitutively the Foxp3 transcription factor [33].

As well as in *T. crassiceps* infection, during NCC a period of immunosuppression has been reported. One study extracting polymorphonuclear (PMN) cells from 11 patients diagnosed with NCC, showed a clear immunosuppression in response to TsES antigens from the scolex of *T. solium*, also NCC patients with calcified cysts displayed increased immunosuppression [34]. The same study showed the suppressor capacity of TsES, completely inhibiting the proliferative response to mitogens like phytohaemagglutinin (PHA) and concanavalin A (ConA) [34]. These results are different to those published by a different research group, under the same conditions, where NCC patients without treatment did not show differences in the percentages of CD3$^+$, CD4$^+$ and CD8$^+$ T cell populations. Moreover, blood cells from these NCC patients showed the same proliferative capacity to ConA or crude *T. solium* antigens compared with controls, and finally also PMN cells produced IL-2 [4]. Is not clear what is the correct scenario, maybe another process or data were not considered in the clinical history between these both studies, like age of the patient, sex, or any oncological or immunosuppressive constitutive status. In fact, more recently published data showed that if analyzed groups of patients with NCC are divided by the local site of the infection in either parenchymal (infection is resolved in general) or subarachnoid (increased symptomatology and pathology), the group of patients with subarachnoid infection has an increased immunoregulatory microenvironment characterized by IL-10, TGF-β and expanded Treg cell frequencies *ex-vivo* [35].

3.2 Immune-regulatory myeloid-derived mechanisms

The generation of an immune-regulatory environment could have an effect not exclusively in T cells, but in all immune cells, including all myeloid-derived lineages such as macrophages, dendritic cells (DCs) and PMNs. Thus, myeloid cells are key players in the immune response against cysticercosis. In fact, there is evidence suggesting an increased profile of alternative activated macrophages or

M2 macrophages involved in parasite expulsion and tissue repair during helminth infections, which induce protection to the host [36]. However, in cysticercosis, the scenario appears to be different.

During *T. crassiceps* infection it was suggested that recruited $CD11b^{+}Gr1^{+}$ myeloid-derived suppressor cells (MDSCs) impaired the T cell proliferation by secretion of high amounts of nitric oxide (NO) at early stages of an intraperitoneal infection. This classic inflammatory activation is switched at chronic stages, where $CD11b^{+}Gr1^{+}$ cells express arginase, YM-1 and FIZZ1 genes, associated with an M2 phenotype (**Figure 1**). This immunosuppressive microenvironment favors IL-4 and IL-13 production, expanding the MDSCs population and also, inducing lipid mediators' activation like 13-hydroxyoctadecadienoic acid and 15-hydroxyeicosatetraenoic acid, associated with the immunosuppression of T cell proliferation [37]. Also, alternative-activated macrophages (AAMs or M2) from chronic *T. crassiceps* infection have the ability to produce high levels of IL-6 and Prostaglandin E2 (see below), reducing the proliferative capacity of $CD4^{+}$ T cells in a STAT-6 dependent-pathway (**Figure 1**) [11], suggesting that AAMs are necessaries to induce the permissive microenvironment for the colonization of *T. crassiceps* infection. In fact, it was demonstrated that an early in vivo depletion of AAMs by using clodronate liposomes, increases the resistance against *T. crassiceps* [38], making stronger the hypothesis that experimental cysticercosis has an AAMs-dependence for a successful infection. Later, it was shown that these AAMs induce anergy on $CD4^{+}$ T cells during *T. crassiceps* infection, and that such an event depends on PDL1 and PDL2 expression in the surface membrane of AAMs [39].

On the other hand, monocyte-derived DCs co-cultured with CD4 naïve cells in presence of *T. solium* cysticerci promotes both, Treg and DCs cells differentiation towards a tolerogenic profile featured by a higher expression of Signaling Lymphocytic Activation Molecule 1 (SLAM1), B7-H1 and CD205 molecules (**Figure 1**). These results suggest that *T. solium* cysticerci has the ability to induce both Treg cells as well as suppressive or tolerogenic DCs [29].

4. Regulatory mechanisms mediated by cytokines, antibodies, and soluble immune factors

4.1 IL-10

IL-10 is produced by innate cells like myeloid and plasmacytoid DCs and macrophages, and is also produced by Breg cells, Th2, Th17 and Treg cells from the adaptive immune response. This capacity to be produced from several immune cell lineages, depends on the signal pathways activated like ERK, and also from transcription factors like STAT3, STAT4, STAT6 and cytokines like TGF-**β** [40]. One of the main features of IL-10 is its capacity to induce immunosuppression, reducing IL-12 and TNF-a levels. By transcriptomic array analyses, we observed that miR-125a-5p, miR-762, and miR-484 microRNAs, are associated with the targeting of inflammatory profiles of macrophages favoring the IL-10 signaling pathway, suggesting that *T. crassiceps* and its products induce post-transcriptional suppression mechanisms of the immune response [41]. Earlier studies performed in experimental cysticercosis caused by chronical *T. crassiceps* infection, indicated a strong Th2 biased immune response featured by high production of IL-4, IL-6 and IL-13 cytokines as well as increased IL-10 levels [12]. These findings were just recently confirmed by an independent group highlighting the importance of IL-10 cytokine [42].

4.2 Transforming growth factor beta (TGF-β)

TGF-β is a cytokine involved in some situations during immune and not immune phenomena. It has a role in the control of cell proliferation and differentiation of some cell types like either Treg or Th17 cells [43, 44]. Also, by itself, it has the capacity to induce a suppressive environment in scenarios where required, like mucosal immune reactions. Dysregulation of TGF-β generates inflammatory disorders such as spontaneous colitis [45]. In the *T. solium* genome were found some genes homologs with the TGF-β receptor family, including some evolved in its down-stream transduction pathway. In fact, it was confirmed by RT-PCR and western blot assays that cysts of *T. solium* express the type I and type II receptor for TGF- β. Also, the addition of TGF- β to the culture media for both *T. crassiceps* and *T. solium* adequate conditions, promotes both the reproduction of *T. crassiceps* and the survival of *T. solium in vitro*. Finally, high levels of TGF-β were found in the cerebrospinal fluid from patients diagnosed with NCC [46]. All these results suggest a strong direct and indirect role for TGF-β in the process of immunosuppression during *T. solium* infection.

4.3 Osteopontin

Osteopontin (OPN) is a Th1 type cytokine upstream of IL-12 that has a role in the granuloma formation in inflamed tissues [47]. It was shown that blood cells co-cultured with TsES or viable cysticerci from *T. solium* led to decreased levels of OPN, IL-12 and IFN-γ. Injection of recombinant OPN into tissues surrounding implanted cysticerci enhances inflammatory responses, which suggests that TsES may have molecules that block OPN activity as a target for immunosuppression [48].

4.4 Antibodies

Humoral immune response has been described for its essential role against helminth infections, being IgE antibody isotype a cornerstone to induce protection [49]. However, during taeniasis and cysticercosis, little information about the role of B cells has been described. It was shown that an antibody called anti-GK-1 (IgG) obtained from the serum of pigs infected with *T. solium*, has an epitope shared by both *T. crassiceps* and *T. solium* [50] and also, has the capacity to inhibit the development of *T. solium* cysticerci into adult stage by recognition of the cyst protein KE7 [51]. This protective role for anti-GK1 antibodies is complement-mediated during *T. solium* infection [50, 52]. However, these results are the only data obtained for humoral immune response during taeniasis and cysticercosis. During experimental cysticercosis and during NCC, is clear that immunosuppression favors the establishment of the parasite, and this GK-1 antibody-mediated mechanism has naturally no success; maybe a molecule of the parasite has the capacity to inhibit this protective function, which in turn induces immunosuppression. Is necessary to clarify this point with specific and deeper experiments.

4.5 Prostaglandin E2

Some lipids from eicosanoid family derivatives from arachidonic acid, like prostaglandin E2 (PGE2), have been described as potent immunosuppressant molecules [53]. It has been described that administration *in vivo* of PGE2 in *T. crassiceps* infected mice favors both parasite growth and cytokine production of IL-10 and IL-6 by splenocytes and reduces the proliferative capacity of splenocytes stimulated with ConA. On the other hand, the administration of indomethacin, an inhibitor of PGE2 synthesis, induced the reduction of both the parasite growth and cytokine production of IL-10 and IL-6, increasing the ConA-proliferative response of splenocytes (**Figure 1**) [54]. These results suggest that *T. crassiceps* can induce the production of PGE2 indirectly from some cellular types, like almost all cells of the host, as a mechanism of immunoregulation [54]. Also, it is possible that some molecules from TcES could be a similar biomolecule like PGE2, mimicking their function and directly inducing immunosuppression, like the TGF-β phenomenon observed during *T. solium* infection.

5. Immunoregulation mediated by Taenia-derived products

5.1 Paramyosin

Paramyosin is an α-helical coiled coil 100 KDa protein that is present in muscle and tegument of the larval stage of *T. solium* [55]. This protein can bind to the protein C1q of the complement, therefore, inhibiting the complement cascade [56]. This was the first evasive mechanism described for this parasite. Vaccine strategies performed to block the activity of this protein resulted in almost 80% of protection [57].

5.2 Glutathione transferase

Glutathione transferase (GST) is an essential enzyme in the metabolism of cestodes, mainly for the detoxification of xenobiotics, it is localized on the cysticerci tegument of *T. solium* [58]. This molecule appears to have a immunomodulatory role given that its use as a putative vaccine was able to reduce parasite load on experimental cysticercosis, mainly by activating macrophages to produce pro-inflammatory cytokines [59]. These data indicate that *T. solium* and *T. crassiceps* may have pro and anti-inflammatory mixed molecules.

5.3 TcES or TsES antigens

Analysis of *T. solium* excreted/secreted antigens (TsES) showed a cysteine protease activity for these molecules, having the capacity to induce apoptosis specifically in $CD4^+$ but no in $CD8^+$ T cells, which is evidence of a direct mode of immunosuppression over a population of the immune response (**Figure 1**). Cocultured cysts of *T. solium* with lymphocytes *in vitro* have not the same effect to induce apoptosis like TsES [60]. Also, it was suggested that natural infection of pigs with *T. solium* cysticerci recruits $CD3^+$ cells to the brain which are killed by apoptosis [61].

Studies in our laboratory demonstrated that TcES products have the capacity to block TLR4 and TLR9 initial signaling pathway in DCs, which has a negative effect over their maturation, their production of pro-inflammatory cytokines and also, to induce alloreactive T cell proliferation, but in an IL-10 independent pathway. All these regulatory effects were carbohydrate-dependent in the TcES, because the chemical alteration of glycans switch this tolerogenic environment to one favoring DCs maturation and secretion of pro-inflammatory cytokines (**Figure 1**) such as IL-12 and TNF-α [62]. Moreover, it was shown that the *in vivo* treatment with TcES, has the capacity to induce the differentiation of monocytes to AAMs expressing PDL1 and PDL2, which in turn down-modulate the activity of experimental autoimmune encephalomyelitis EAE [63]. Furthermore, it was shown that in the murine model of NCC with the helminth *Mesocestoides corti*, the inhibition of TLR-initiated regulation of inflammatory cytokines exists. This effect is caused by an inhibition of acetylation and phosphorylation of both NF-kB and JNK which causes an accumulation of Ca^{2+} in the endoplasmic reticulum [22]. Probably, this phenomenon is similarly used by *T. solium* during initial establishment of the infection, however, deeper research is necessary in this field (**Figure 1**).

Also, it was shown that the nature of antigens of *T. solium* is essential to induce a proper immune response. Within *T. solium* crude lysate antigen, cyst wall antigen, and cyst fluid antigen, only low molecular weight fractions of cyst fluid are immunodominant, with the capacity to induce the production of inflammatory cytokines, but mainly higher levels of IL-10 and IL-4 by stimulated lymphocytes of patients with NCC [64]. Besides, it was suggested that the time of TcES obtention has a different impact over the kind of immunosuppression observed; TcES obtained early in infection, suppress the proliferative response of splenocytes stimulated with ConA than TcES obtained late in infection. Also, these early obtained TcES suppress the production of IFN-γ and IL-4 efficiently [65].

6. Conclusions

It has been largely known that helminthic infections induce strong Th2-mediated immune responses associated with regulation of inflammatory responses. Here, it has been described the different molecules and pathways altered by *T. solium* and *T. crassiceps* infection. Is noteworthy that some clinical studies point out that this immunomodulation favors both the parasite and host survival when the parasite is allocated in the brain, mainly because the inflammatory response is inhibited, avoiding the damage expected from a strong inflammatory response.

The anti-inflammatory activities and immunoregulatory properties found in both *T. solium* and *T. crassiceps* parasites and their products, can be useful beyond the host–parasite interactions. During some allergic diseases like asthma and rhinitis, the hygiene hypothesis has strengthened the idea of the historical necessity to down-modulate the immune response by mechanisms of natural coevolution, like the infection with helminth parasites [66]. In the same order of ideas, because of all these suppressive capacities of both *T. crassiceps* parasites and their TcES molecules, we hypothesized that it probably has the capacity to modulate chronic diseases associated with inflammation. We observed a clear role of both *T. crassiceps* and their TcES antigens in the modulation of experimental autoimmune encephalomyelitis (EAE) [67, 68], colitis-associated colon cancer (CAC) [69, 70], experimental colitis [71] and type 1 diabetes [72].

Lately, we have observed that the mechanisms used by the parasites that cause infectious diseases, such as taeniasis and cysticercosis, are very similar processes, and we dare to suggest that they are the same, to those occurring during the main oncological (solid) pathologies. The fact that a carcinogenic transformed cell induces an immunosuppressive process through immune-checkpoints such as PD1, CTLA-4 or Tim3, is a mechanism that had already been described in the past, during cysticercosis. So, immunoregulation and immunosuppression are natural selection mechanisms that pathogens take advantage of to be able to survive in a hostile environment and turn it to favor them, to face a variety of processes of continuous and varied attack of the immune response. Therefore, understanding and deciphering the why, how, and when these natural selection processes occur, we will be able to apply the lesson obtained during infectious diseases in processes affecting the current public health, like the main oncological pathologies.

Acknowledgements

"This work was supported by CONACYT grant number A1-S-37879 and DGAPA-PAPIIT-UNAM grants numbers IA209720 and IN226519.

Conflict of interest

"The authors declare no conflict of interest."

Abbreviations

AAM	Alternatively activated macrophages
ConA	Concanavalin A
CTLA-4	Cytotoxic T-Lymphocyte Antigen 4
DCs	Dendritic cells
DPI	Days post-infection
EAE	Experimental autoimmune encephalomyelitis
ELISA	Enzyme-linked Immuno Assay
ERK	Extracellular signal regulated kinases
Foxp3	Forkhead box P3 transcription factor
FIZZ1	Found in inflammatory zone 1 gene
Gal-9	Galectin-9
Gal-7	Galectin-7
IFN-γ	Interferon-gamma
IgE	Immunoglobulin E
IgG	Immunoglobulin G
IL-2	Interleukin-2
IL-4	Interleukin-4
IL4Rα	Interleukin4 receptor α
IL-6	Interleukin-6
IL-10	Interleukin-10
IL-12	Interleukin-12
IL-13	Interleukin-13
IP	Intraperitoneal
MDSC	Myeloid-derived suppressor cells
NCC	Neurocysticercosis
NCS	Nervous Central System
NO	Nitric oxide
OPN	Osteopontin
PD1	Programmed death 1
PDL1	Programmed Death-ligand 1
PDL2	Programmed Death-ligand 2
PGE2	Prostaglandin E2
PHA	phytohaemagglutinin
PMN	Polymorphonuclear cells
RT-PCR	Real time polymerase chain reaction
SLAMF1	Signaling Lymphocytic Activation Molecule 1
STAT3	Signal transducer and activator of transcription 3
STAT4	Signal transducer and activator of transcription 4
STAT6	Signal transducer and activator of transcription 6
TcES	*Taenia crassiceps* excreted/secreted antigens

TGF-β	Tumor growth factor beta
TNF-α	Tumor Necrosis Factor Alpha
Th1	T helper cells 1
Th2	T helper cells 2
Th17	T helper cells 17
Tim3	T-cell Immunoglobulin domain and Mucin domain 3
TLR4	Toll-like receptor 4
TLR9	Toll-like receptor 4
Treg	Regulatory T cells
Tr1	T regulatory Type 1 population
TsES	*Taenia solium* excreted/secreted antigens

Author details

Jonadab E. Olguín[1,2] and Luis Ignacio Terrazas[1,2*]

1 Laboratorio Nacional en Salud: Diagnóstico Molecular y Efecto Ambiental en Enfermedades Crónico-degenerativas, Facultad de Estudios Superiores Iztacala, Universidad Nacional Autónoma de México (UNAM), Mexico

2 Unidad de Biomedicina, Facultad de Estudios Superiores Iztacala, UNAM, Mexico

*Address all correspondence to: literrazas@unam.mx

References

[1] Gonzales I, Rivera JT, Garcia HH, Cysticercosis Working Group in P. Pathogenesis of Taenia solium taeniasis and cysticercosis. Parasite immunology. 2016;38:136-146. DOI: 10.1111/pim. 12307

[2] Garcia HH, Nash TE, Del Brutto OH. Clinical symptoms, diagnosis, and treatment of neurocysticercosis. The Lancet Neurology. 2014;13:1202-1215. DOI: 10.1016/S1474-4422(14)70094-8

[3] Flisser A, Correa D. Neuro cysticercosis may no longer be a public health problem in Mexico. PLoS neglected tropical diseases. 2010;4:e831. DOI: 10.1371/journal.pntd.0000831

[4] Medina-Escutia E, Morales-Lopez Z, Proano JV, Vazquez J, Bermudez V, Navarrete VO, et al. Cellular immune response and Th1/Th2 cytokines in human neurocysticercosis: lack of immune suppression. The Journal of parasitology. 2001;87:587-590. DOI: 10.1645/0022-3395(2001)087[0587,CIR ATT]2.0.CO;2

[5] Ito A, Plancarte A, Ma L, Kong Y, Flisser A, Cho SY, et al. Novel antigens for neurocysticercosis: simple method for preparation and evaluation for serodiagnosis. The American journal of tropical medicine and hygiene. 1998;59:291-294. DOI: 10.4269/ ajtmh.1998.59.291

[6] Avila G, Teran N, Aguilar-Vega L, Maravilla P, Mata-Miranda P, Flisser A. Laboratory animal models for human Taenia solium. Parasitology international. 2006;55 Suppl:S99-S103. DOI: 10.1016/j.parint.2005.11.015

[7] Maravilla P, Garza-Rodriguez A, Gomez-Diaz B, Jimenez-Gonzalez DE, Toral-Bastida E, Martinez-Ocana J, et al. Chinchilla laniger can be used as an experimental model for Taenia solium taeniasis. Parasitology international. 2011;60:364-370. DOI: 10.1016/j. parint.2011.06.002

[8] Willms K, Zurabian R. Taenia crassiceps: in vivo and in vitro models. Parasitology. 2010;137:335-346. DOI: 10.1017/S0031182009991442

[9] Dorais FJ, Esch GW. Growth rate of two Taenia crassiceps strains. Experimental parasitology. 1969;25: 395-398. DOI: 10.1016/0014-4894(69) 90086-1

[10] Lopez-Briones S, Lamoyi E, Fragoso G, Soloski MJ, Sciutto E. Taenia crassiceps cysticercosis: immune response in susceptible and resistant BALB/c mouse substrains. Parasitology research. 2003;90:236-242. DOI: 10.1007/s00436-003-0848-z

[11] Rodriguez-Sosa M, Satoskar AR, Calderon R, Gomez-Garcia L, Saavedra R, Bojalil R, et al. Chronic helminth infection induces alternatively activated macrophages expressing high levels of CCR5 with low interleukin-12 production and Th2-biasing ability. Infection and immunity. 2002;70:3656-3664. DOI: 10.1128/iai.70.7.3656-3664. 2002

[12] Terrazas LI, Bojalil R, Govezensky T, Larralde C. Shift from an early protective Th1-type immune response to a late permissive Th2-type response in murine cysticercosis (Taenia crassiceps). The Journal of parasitology. 1998;84:74-81. DOI:

[13] Rodriguez-Sosa M, David JR, Bojalil R, Satoskar AR, Terrazas LI. Cutting edge: susceptibility to the larval stage of the helminth parasite Taenia crassiceps is mediated by Th2 response induced via STAT6 signaling. Journal of immunology. 2002;168:3135-3139. DOI: 10.4049/jimmunol.168.7.3135

[14] Terrazas LI, Cruz M, Rodriguez-Sosa M, Bojalil R, Garcia-Tamayo F, Larralde C. Th1-type cytokines improve resistance to murine cysticercosis caused by Taenia crassiceps. Parasitology research. 1999;85:135-141. DOI: 10.1007/s004360050522

[15] Toenjes SA, Spolski RJ, Mooney KA, Kuhn RE. gamma delta T cells do not play a major role in controlling infection in experimental cysticercosis. Parasitology. 1999;119 (Pt 4):413-418. DOI: 10.1017/s0031182099004771

[16] Vaidya A, Singhal S, Dhall S, Manohar A, Mahajan H. Asymptomatic disseminated cysticercosis. Journal of clinical and diagnostic research : JCDR. 2013;7:1761-1763. DOI: 10.7860/JCDR/2013/5465.3269

[17] Herrick JA, Maharathi B, Kim JS, Abundis GG, Garg A, Gonzales I, et al. Inflammation is a key risk factor for persistent seizures in neurocysticercosis. Annals of clinical and translational neurology. 2018;5:630-639. DOI: 10.1002/acn3.562

[18] Naveed M, Zhou QG, Xu C, Taleb A, Meng F, Ahmed B, et al. Gut-brain axis: A matter of concern in neuropsychiatric disorders...! Progress in neuro-psychopharmacology & biological psychiatry. 2021;104:110051. DOI: 10.1016/j.pnpbp.2020.110051

[19] Donskow-Lysoniewska K, Maruszewska-Cheruiyot M, Stear M. The interaction of host and nematode galectins influences the outcome of gastrointestinal nematode infections. Parasitology. 2021;148:648-654. DOI: 10.1017/S003118202100007X

[20] Gieseck RL, 3rd, Wilson MS, Wynn TA. Type 2 immunity in tissue repair and fibrosis. Nature reviews Immunology. 2018;18:62-76. DOI: 10.1038/nri.2017.90

[21] Walker JA, McKenzie ANJ. TH2 cell development and function. Nature reviews Immunology. 2018;18:121-133. DOI: 10.1038/nri.2017.118

[22] Sun Y, Chauhan A, Sukumaran P, Sharma J, Singh BB, Mishra BB. Inhibition of store-operated calcium entry in microglia by helminth factors: implications for immune suppression in neurocysticercosis. Journal of neuroinflammation. 2014;11:210. DOI: 10.1186/s12974-014-0210-7

[23] McLeod R, Eisenhauer P, Mack D, Brown C, Filice G, Spitalny G. Immune responses associated with early survival after peroral infection with Toxoplasma gondii. Journal of immunology 1989;142:3247-3255. DOI:

[24] Salinas N, Olguin JE, Castellanos C, Saavedra R. T cell suppression in vitro during Toxoplasma gondii infection is the result of IL-2 competition between Tregs and T cells leading to death of proliferating T cells. Scandinavian journal of immunology. 2014;79:1-11. DOI: 10.1111/sji.12120

[25] Pereira WF, Ribeiro-Gomes FL, Guillermo LV, Vellozo NS, Montalvao F, Dosreis GA, et al. Myeloid-derived suppressor cells help protective immunity to Leishmania major infection despite suppressed T cell responses. Journal of leukocyte biology. 2011;90:1191-1197. DOI: 10.1189/jlb.1110608

[26] Sztein MB, Kierszenbaum F. Suppression by Trypanosoma cruzi of T-cell receptor expression by activated human lymphocytes. Immunology. 1992;77:277-283. DOI:

[27] Zepeda N, Solano S, Copitin N, Fernandez AM, Hernandez L, Tato P, et al. Decrease of peritoneal inflammatory CD4(+), CD8(+), CD19(+) lymphocytes and apoptosis of eosinophils in a murine Taenia crassiceps infection. Parasitology

research. 2010;107:1129-1135. DOI: 10.1007/s00436-010-1980-1

[28] Spolski RJ, Alexander-Miller MA, Kuhn RE. Suppressed cytotoxic T lymphocyte responses in experimental cysticercosis. Veterinary parasitology. 2002;106:325-330. DOI: 10.1016/s0304-4017(02)00105-x

[29] Adalid-Peralta L, Arce-Sillas A, Fragoso G, Cardenas G, Rosetti M, Casanova-Hernandez D, et al. Cysticerci drive dendritic cells to promote in vitro and in vivo Tregs differentiation. Clinical & developmental immunology. 2013;2013:981468. DOI: 10.1155/2013/981468

[30] Arce-Sillas A, Alvarez-Luquin DD, Cardenas G, Casanova-Hernandez D, Fragoso G, Hernandez M, et al. Interleukin 10 and dendritic cells are the main suppression mediators of regulatory T cells in human neurocysticercosis. Clinical and experimental immunology. 2016;183:271-279. DOI: 10.1111/cei.12709

[31] de Ruiter K, Jochems SP, Tahapary DL, Stam KA, Konig M, van Unen V, et al. Helminth infections drive heterogeneity in human type 2 and regulatory cells. Science translational medicine. 2020;12. DOI: 10.1126/scitranslmed.aaw3703

[32] Gagliani N, Magnani CF, Huber S, Gianolini ME, Pala M, Licona-Limon P, et al. Coexpression of CD49b and LAG-3 identifies human and mouse T regulatory type 1 cells. Nature medicine. 2013;19:739-746. DOI: 10.1038/nm.3179

[33] Olguin JE, Medina-Andrade I, Rodriguez T, Rodriguez-Sosa M, Terrazas LI. Relevance of Regulatory T Cells during Colorectal Cancer Development. Cancers. 2020;12. DOI: 10.3390/cancers12071888

[34] Bueno EC, Vaz AJ, Machado LR, Livramento JA, Avila SL, Ferreira AW. Antigen-specific suppression of cultured lymphocytes from patients with neurocysticercosis. Clinical and experimental immunology. 2001;126:304-310. DOI: 10.1046/j.1365-2249.2001.01579.x

[35] Tuero I, Palma S, Cabeza F, Saleemi S, Rodriguez S, Gonzales I, et al. A Comparative Study of Peripheral Immune Responses to Taenia solium in Individuals with Parenchymal and Subarachnoid Neurocysticercosis. PLoS neglected tropical diseases. 2015;9:e0004143. DOI: 10.1371/journal.pntd.0004143

[36] Coakley G, Harris NL. Interactions between macrophages and helminths. Parasite immunology. 2020;42:e12717. DOI: 10.1111/pim.12717

[37] Brys L, Beschin A, Raes G, Ghassabeh GH, Noel W, Brandt J, et al. Reactive oxygen species and 12/15-lipoxygenase contribute to the antiproliferative capacity of alternatively activated myeloid cells elicited during helminth infection. Journal of immunology. 2005;174:6095-6104. DOI: 10.4049/jimmunol.174.10.6095

[38] Reyes JL, Terrazas CA, Alonso-Trujillo J, van Rooijen N, Satoskar AR, Terrazas LI. Early removal of alternatively activated macrophages leads to Taenia crassiceps cysticercosis clearance in vivo. International journal for parasitology. 2010;40:731-742. DOI: 10.1016/j.ijpara.2009.11.014

[39] Terrazas LI, Montero D, Terrazas CA, Reyes JL, Rodriguez-Sosa M. Role of the programmed Death-1 pathway in the suppressive activity of alternatively activated macrophages in experimental cysticercosis. International journal for parasitology. 2005;35:1349-1358. DOI: 10.1016/j.ijpara.2005.06.003

[40] Saraiva M, O'Garra A. The regulation of IL-10 production by

immune cells. Nature reviews Immunology. 2010;10:170-181. DOI: 10.1038/nri2711

[41] Martinez-Saucedo D, Ruiz-Rosado JD, Terrazas C, Callejas BE, Satoskar AR, Partida-Sanchez S, et al. Taenia crassiceps-Excreted/Secreted Products Induce a Defined MicroRNA Profile that Modulates Inflammatory Properties of Macrophages. Journal of immunology research. 2019;2019:2946713. DOI: 10.1155/2019/2946713

[42] Diaz-Zaragoza M, Jimenez L, Hernandez M, Hernandez-Avila R, Navarro L, Ochoa-Sanchez A, et al. Protein expression profile of Taenia crassiceps cysticerci related to Th1- and Th2-type responses in the mouse cysticercosis model. Acta tropica. 2020;212:105696. DOI: 10.1016/j.actatropica.2020.105696

[43] Morikawa M, Derynck R, Miyazono K. TGF-beta and the TGF-beta Family: Context-Dependent Roles in Cell and Tissue Physiology. Cold Spring Harbor perspectives in biology. 2016;8. DOI: 10.1101/cshperspect.a021873

[44] Lee GR. The Balance of Th17 versus Treg Cells in Autoimmunity. International journal of molecular sciences. 2018;19. DOI: 10.3390/ijms19030730

[45] Ihara S, Hirata Y, Koike K. TGF-beta in inflammatory bowel disease: a key regulator of immune cells, epithelium, and the intestinal microbiota. Journal of gastroenterology. 2017;52:777-787. DOI: 10.1007/s00535-017-1350-1

[46] Adalid-Peralta L, Rosas G, Arce-Sillas A, Bobes RJ, Cardenas G, Hernandez M, et al. Effect of Transforming Growth Factor-beta upon Taenia solium and Taenia crassiceps Cysticerci. Scientific reports. 2017;7:12345. DOI: 10.1038/s41598-017-12202-z

[47] Ashkar S, Weber GF, Panoutsakopoulou V, Sanchirico ME, Jansson M, Zawaideh S, et al. Eta-1 (osteopontin): an early component of type-1 (cell-mediated) immunity. Science. 2000;287:860-864. DOI: 10.1126/science.287.5454.860

[48] Wang IC, Fan PC, Lu SC, Fan CK, Su KE. Suppression of host Th1-type granulomatous inflammation by Taenia solium metacestodes is related to down-regulation of osteopontin gene expression. International journal for parasitology. 2008;38:239-248. DOI: 10.1016/j.ijpara.2007.07.010

[49] Wu LC, Zarrin AA. The production and regulation of IgE by the immune system. Nature reviews Immunology. 2014;14:247-259. DOI: 10.1038/nri3632

[50] Garcia G, Sciutto E, Fragoso G, Cruz-Revilla C, Toledo A, Villalobos N, et al. Inhibitory role of antibodies in the development of Taenia solium and Taenia crassiceps toward reproductive and pathogenic stages. The Journal of parasitology. 2001;87:582-586. DOI: 10.1645/0022-3395(2001)087[0582,IROAIT]2.0.CO;2

[51] Bobes RJ, Navarrete-Perea J, Ochoa-Leyva A, Anaya VH, Hernandez M, Cervantes-Torres J, et al. Experimental and Theoretical Approaches To Investigate the Immunogenicity of Taenia solium-Derived KE7 Antigen. Infection and immunity. 2017;85. DOI: 10.1128/IAI.00395-17

[52] Nunez G, Villalobos N, Herrera CP, Navarrete-Perea J, Mendez A, Martinez-Maya JJ, et al. Anti-GK1 antibodies damage Taenia crassiceps cysticerci through complement activation. Parasitology research. 2018;117:2543-2553. DOI: 10.1007/s00436-018-5943-2

[53] Park JY, Pillinger MH, Abramson SB. Prostaglandin E2

synthesis and secretion: the role of PGE2 synthases. Clinical immunology. 2006;119:229-240. DOI: 10.1016/j.clim.2006.01.016

[54] Terrazas LI, Bojalil R, Rodriguez-Sosa M, Govezensky T, Larralde C. Taenia crassiceps cysticercosis: a role for prostaglandin E2 in susceptibility. Parasitology research. 1999;85:1025-1031. DOI: 10.1007/s004360050676

[55] Laclette JP, Landa A, Arcos L, Willms K, Davis AE, Shoemaker CB. Paramyosin is the Schistosoma mansoni (Trematoda) homologue of antigen B from Taenia solium (Cestoda). Molecular and biochemical parasitology. 1991;44:287-295. DOI: 10.1016/0166-6851(91)90015-x

[56] Laclette JP, Shoemaker CB, Richter D, Arcos L, Pante N, Cohen C, et al. Paramyosin inhibits complement C1. Journal of immunology. 1992;148: 124-128. DOI:

[57] Vargas-Parada L, Laclette JP. Gene structure of Taenia solium paramyosin. Parasitology research. 2003;89:375-378. DOI: 10.1007/s00436-002-0761-x

[58] Vibanco-Perez N, Jimenez L, Merchant MT, Landa A. Characterization of glutathione S-transferase of Taenia solium. The Journal of parasitology. 1999;85:448-453. DOI:

[59] Vega-Angeles VT, Terrazas LI, Ledesma-Soto Y, Jimenez L, Landa A. Taenia solium glutathione transferase fraction activates macrophages and favors the development of Th1-type response. Bioscience reports. 2019;39. DOI: 10.1042/BSR20181132

[60] Tato P, Fernandez AM, Solano S, Borgonio V, Garrido E, Sepulveda J, et al. A cysteine protease from Taenia solium metacestodes induce apoptosis in human CD4+ T-cells. Parasitology research. 2004;92:197-204. DOI: 10.1007/s00436-003-1008-1

[61] Sikasunge CS, Phiri IK, Johansen MV, Willingham AL, 3rd, Leifsson PS. Host-cell apoptosis in Taenia solium-induced brain granulomas in naturally infected pigs. Parasitology. 2008;135:1237-1242. DOI: 10.1017/S0031182008004678

[62] Terrazas CA, Gomez-Garcia L, Terrazas LI. Impaired pro-inflammatory cytokine production and increased Th2-biasing ability of dendritic cells exposed to Taenia excreted/secreted antigens: A critical role for carbohydrates but not for STAT6 signaling. International journal for parasitology. 2010;40:1051-1062. DOI: 10.1016/j.ijpara.2010.02.016

[63] Terrazas C, de Dios Ruiz-Rosado J, Amici SA, Jablonski KA, Martinez-Saucedo D, Webb LM, et al. Helminth-induced Ly6C(hi) monocyte-derived alternatively activated macrophages suppress experimental autoimmune encephalomyelitis. Scientific reports. 2017;7:40814. DOI: 10.1038/srep40814

[64] Amit P, Prasad KN, Kumar GR, Shweta T, Sanjeev J, Kumar PV, et al. Immune response to different fractions of Taenia solium cyst fluid antigens in patients with neurocysticercosis. Experimental parasitology. 2011;127:687-692. DOI: 10.1016/j.exppara.2010.11.006

[65] Spolski RJ, Corson J, Thomas PG, Kuhn RE. Parasite-secreted products regulate the host response to larval Taenia crassiceps. Parasite immunology. 2000;22:297-305. DOI: 10.1046/j.1365-3024.2000.00301.x

[66] Logan J, Navarro S, Loukas A, Giacomin P. Helminth-induced regulatory T cells and suppression of allergic responses. Current opinion in immunology. 2018;54:1-6. DOI: 10.1016/j.coi.2018.05.007

[67] Peon AN, Ledesma-Soto Y, Olguin JE, Bautista-Donis M, Sciutto E, Terrazas LI. Helminth Products Potently Modulate Experimental Autoimmune Encephalomyelitis by Downregulating Neuroinflammation and Promoting a Suppressive Microenvironment. Mediators of inflammation. 2017;2017:8494572. DOI: 10.1155/2017/8494572

[68] Reyes JL, Espinoza-Jimenez AF, Gonzalez MI, Verdin L, Terrazas LI. Taenia crassiceps infection abrogates experimental autoimmune encephalomyelitis. Cellular immunology. 2011;267:77-87. DOI: 10.1016/j.cellimm.2010.11.006

[69] Callejas BE, Mendoza-Rodriguez MG, Villamar-Cruz O, Reyes-Martinez S, Sanchez-Barrera CA, Rodriguez-Sosa M, et al. Helminth-derived molecules inhibit colitis-associated colon cancer development through NF-kappaB and STAT3 regulation. International journal of cancer. 2019;145:3126-3139. DOI: 10.1002/ijc.32626

[70] Leon-Cabrera S, Callejas BE, Ledesma-Soto Y, Coronel J, Perez-Plasencia C, Gutierrez-Cirlos EB, et al. Extraintestinal helminth infection reduces the development of colitis-associated tumorigenesis. International journal of biological sciences. 2014;10:948-956. DOI: 10.7150/ijbs.9033

[71] Ledesma-Soto Y, Callejas BE, Terrazas CA, Reyes JL, Espinoza-Jimenez A, Gonzalez MI, et al. Extraintestinal Helminth Infection Limits Pathology and Proinflammatory Cytokine Expression during DSS-Induced Ulcerative Colitis: A Role for Alternatively Activated Macrophages and Prostaglandins. BioMed research international. 2015;2015:563425. DOI: 10.1155/2015/563425

[72] Espinoza-Jimenez A, De Haro R, Terrazas LI. Taenia crassiceps Antigens Control Experimental Type 1 Diabetes by Inducing Alternatively Activated Macrophages. Mediators of inflammation. 2017;2017:8074329. DOI: 10.1155/2017/8074329

Chapter 4

The Long Road to the Immunodiagnosis of Neurocysticercosis: Controversies and Confusions

Marcela Esquivel-Velázquez, Carlos Larralde, Pedro Ostoa-Saloma, Víctor Hugo Del Río Araiza and Jorge Morales-Montor

Abstract

To date, even widely studied, there is not a standard diagnostic method to detect neurocysticercotic patients. The later due to the complex nature of cysticercosis disease and the simplicity of common immunological assumptions involved in explaining the low scores and reproducibility of immunotests in the diagnosis of neurocysticercosis. To begin with, the few studies dealing with the immune response during neurocysticercosis are not conclusive, which of course it is crucial to develop an immunodiagnostic test. Their full recognition should clear confusion and reduce controversy as well as provide avenues of research and technological design. In here, logical arguments add that even under common immunological assumptions, serology of neurocysticercosis will always include false negative and positive results. Thus, serology is no strong support for medical diagnosis of neurocysticercosis (NC). In contrast, immunotests performed in the cerebrospinal fluid (CSF) of neurological patients should have fewer false positive and fewer false negatives than in serum. To conclude, it is argued that high scores in serology for NC will not yield to usual approaches and that success needs of a concerted world-wide effort. A more punctilious strategy based on the design of panels of confirmed positive and negative sera needs to be construed, shared and tested by all interested groups to obtain comparable results. The identification of a set of specific and representative antigens of *Taenia solium* (*T. solium*) and a thorough compilation of the many forms of antibody response of humans to the many forms of *T. solium* disease are also to be considered as one of the most importants factors to the disease.

Keywords: Cysticercosis, Neglected Diseases, Neurocysticercosis, Immunodiagnosis

1. Introduction

Neurocysticercosis (NC) is a disease caused by the larvae (or cysticerci) of the intestinal parasite *Taenia solium* (*T. solium*) when the cysticerci lodges in the central nervous system (CNS). It is considered one of the most important parasitic disease of the CNS [1–3]. Cysticerci may infect humans and may also locate elsewhere of CNS, in skeletal muscles, heart, eyes, diaphragm, tongue and subcutaneous tissues, causing a condition simply referred to as cysticercosis. Cysticerci develop in humans and also in pigs from eggs produced by the adult tapeworm living in the intestine of humans and shed to the environment upon defecation, thus contaminating soil, waters and food.

The most serious condition of *T. solium* disease affecting human health is NC. An estimated 60% of NC cases are non-symptomatic [4], while the rest are symptomatic and exhibit a wide variety of neurological symptoms, being chronic epilepsy and headache the most noticeable [4–6]. Severe forms of NC develop meningitis, encephalitis, arteritis, areas of cerebral infarction and gliosis, as well as anatomical distortion and compression of intracranial structures causing blockade in the flow of cerebrospinal-fluid (CSF) [5–7], frequently leading to endo-cranial hypertension and requiring specialized medical attention and/or surgery to derive CSF and/or remove the parasite. The severe forms of NC seriously impair the patients´ health and may lead to death. Medical diagnosis of NC is impossible on clinical data alone as it presents a variety of nonspecific symptoms [8], while confirmatory diagnosis is established by biopsy, cranial CAT-scans and/or cranial NMR images showing nodular lesions of the brain usually suffice in most cases.

Immunodiagnosis of NC (IDxNC) has long been sought because of the disease's prolonged silent or ambiguous clinical pictures and also because of the low accessibility and impossibly high costs of CAT-scans and NMR-images in endemic countries [1, 9–11]. Not only an effective IDxNC would be a most practical way to facilitate medical diagnosis for millions of poor people in endemic countries, it would also supply sero-epidemiological studies with a low-cost indicator of prevalence of infection. In addition, a positive immune-test would rise the clinical suspicion of early non-symptomatic NC which, if confirmed, would allow to offer early treatment before the parasite does much irreversible CNS damage. Further, simplification of copro-parasitological studies in stools by an immune-test would help to identify carriers of live tapeworms and treat them in order to interrupt transmission in the explosive stage of massive egg production.

Many immunological methods have been tried to detect antibodies and/or antigens of *T. solium* in serum or CSF and feces, and even in urine and saliva [12–16], with variable levels of success in detecting NC cases and tapeworm carriers [17, 18]. The gallery includes *in vitro* tests using complement fixation, precipitation, agglutination, radioimmunoassay and enzyme-based detection systems (ELISA and Western Blots) [8, 19, 20]. Antigens used in diagnosis also vary from whole antigen extracts [14, 21, 22], secreted antigens [23–27], semi-purified fractions and purified natural proteins [6, 12, 16, 28] to recombinant proteins [4, 6, 8–11, 29, 30], and synthetic peptides [31–33], either from *T. solium* or from homologous parasites as *Taenia crassiceps* [2, 13, 19, 21, 32, 34], *Taenia saginata* [22, 35] or *Taenia taeniaeformis* [36]. Most reports initially claim very high specificity/sensitivity scores, sometimes even as high as 100/100%. Enthusiasm soon calms as the methods are applied by different laboratories, in larger numbers of cases and in various epidemiological scenarios of the disease [14, 28, 37, 38]. A sober statement about the state of the art at present times would claim a sensitivity that ranges from 50 to 85% (15–50% false positives) and a specificity of about 80–90% (10--20% false negatives), with large variations within and between tests and low reproducibility between laboratories [14, 28, 38].

2. Generalities of immune response to *Taenia solium* cysticercosis

In recent times it has been found that cysticercosis is importantly driven by the hosts neuroendocrine system function, particularly sex steroid hormones (Morales-Montor and Larralde c, 2005). *Taenia* parasites have developed elaborate mechanisms of interacting with their intermediate hosts. The oncospheres which invade the intermediate host are susceptible to antibody and complement. However, by the time the host has generated an antibody response, the parasites have begun to transform to the more resistant metacestode. The metacestodes have elaborate means of evading complement-mediated destruction, including paramyosin which inhibits C1q, taeniaestatin which inhibits both classical and alternate pathways, and sulfated polysaccharides which activate complement away from the parasite. Similarly, antibody does not seem to be able to kill the mature metacestode. In fact, the parasites may even stimulate the host to produce antibody, which could be bound via Fc receptors and used as a source of protein. Finally, taeniaestatin and other poorly defined factors may interfere with lymphocyte proliferation and macrophage function, thus paralyzing the cellular immune response. Since the symptoms of NC are typically associated with a brisk inflammatory response, we hypothesize that disease is primarily caused by injured or dying parasites. This hypothesis raises important questions in assessing the role of chemotherapy in the management of NC, as well as in the evaluation of clinical trials, most of which were uncontrolled (Morales-Montor et al., 2006).

The generation of protective T cell responses to cysticercosis is a complex process in which cytokines and costimulatory molecules provide signals that direct the development of adaptative immunity (13). The characterization of T cell responses as belonging to either Th1-type responses (dominated by the production of IFN-γ and associated with cell-mediated immunity) or Th2-type responses (characterized by production of IL-4 and IL-5, and associated with humoral immunity) was important because it provided a basis for understanding how T cells contribute to resistance, or susceptibility to cysticercosis (14). Subsequent studies distinguished the role of IL-12 and IL-4 in the development of Th1 and Th2 responses, respectively, but there are other cytokines involved in this process (13). Succintly, it can be sustained that immune response to the worm (adult stage of *T. solium*) is limited to Th2-type mechanisms, while the line of defense against the cysticercus is a mixed

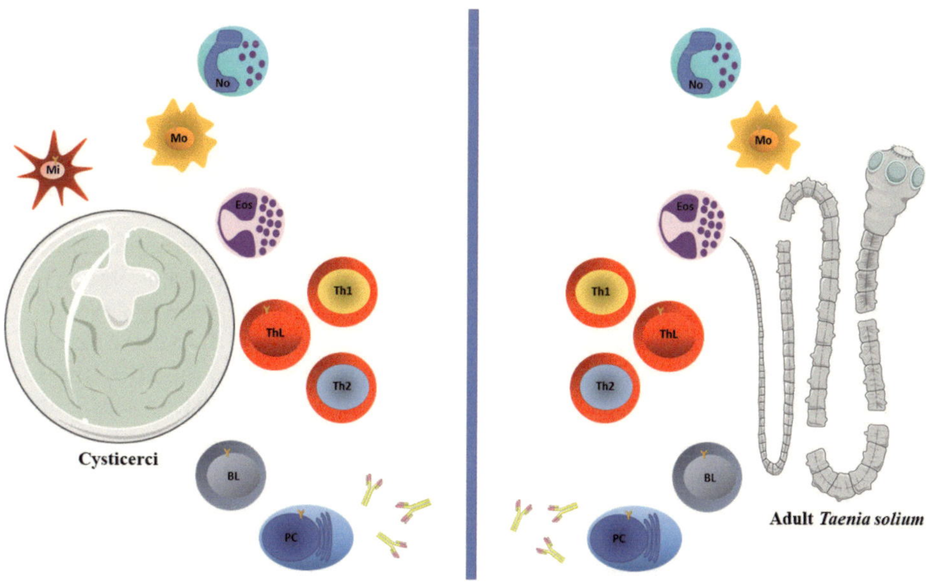

Figure 1.
Cysticerci or adult parasite and associated host immune cells. Mi, microglia/dendritic cell; Mo, macrophage; No, neutrophil; Eos, eosinophil; Th, T helper lymphocyte; Th1, T helper lymphocyte type 1; Th2, T helper lymphocyte type 2; BL, B lymphocyte; PC, plasmatic cell.

Th1-Th2-type immune response, with dominance of Th1-type immune response mechanisms involved in limiting parasite growth and expansion (**Figure 1**).

3. Sources and effects of controversy

Low sensitivity and specificity of IDxNC, as well as variability of results within each method and irregular reproducibility between different laboratories, are cause of discussion and confusion. More than 50 years of insufficiently planned and disaggregated individualistic research using different materials, reagents, techniques and conditions of endemial are involved. Policy of publication favoring alleged breakthroughs tells the luminous half of the stories, creating the false impression that similar results are to be expected by all. The surging of commercial kits and their accompanying propagandistic fanfare has fueled dispute and nurtured distrust because of suspected conflicts of interest without much improvement in diagnostic capacity. The serious problem caused by all this is that the jingle of controversy and confusion has reached medical practice and introduced doubts on the significance of serology in medical diagnosis and epidemiological study surveys. This has in turn retarded the recognition of *T. solium* disease as the great threat it is to human health and the high costs it incurs to public health in endemic countries. It might be of help to clarify the major causes behind the low performance of IDxNC as a preliminary step to reach a consensual agreement on the meaning of its results, its limitations and the ways for improvement.

Low performance and variability are usually thought to rise from the technical virtues or pitfalls of the different available immunological tools and reagents used. There is some reason for argument here but there is much more than that to fully explain the incoherent results and to incorporate in the design of a strategy with a chance of worldwide solid success. Rarely is it recognized faulty results may rise from over-simplified immunological assumptions about this particular host–parasite relationship, incomplete knowledge of the *T. solium* antigen repertoire and/or the immunological complexities derived from the many forms *T solium* has of affecting humans. Because the pleomorphism in *T. solium* disease sets the levels of difficulty for immunological discrimination and is the least recognized cause of controversial results, here we shall describe in somewhat fastidious detail its many different faces.

The exercise illustrates how hard it is the task of immunotests when put to effectively discriminate from the multiple faces of *T solium* disease the one and only of NC. It will also suggest ways of clustering the significant from the insignificant discriminations, for medical as distinguished from epidemiological purposes, as well as point to what is possible and what impossible. Inevitably, some of the major immunological assumptions behind the presence or absence of antibodies and/or antigen in an individual must be dealt-with to some extent since they interact with the disease polymorphism to increment the difficulties of immunodiagnosis for NC. The exercise also explains many of the discrepant findings and should clear some of the controversy as well as point to ways of improvement.

4. The many faces of *T. solium* disease

Any human population under consideration may be divided in two sets according to their having had come in contact with *T. solium* (*I*) or not (*0*) (**Figure 2**).

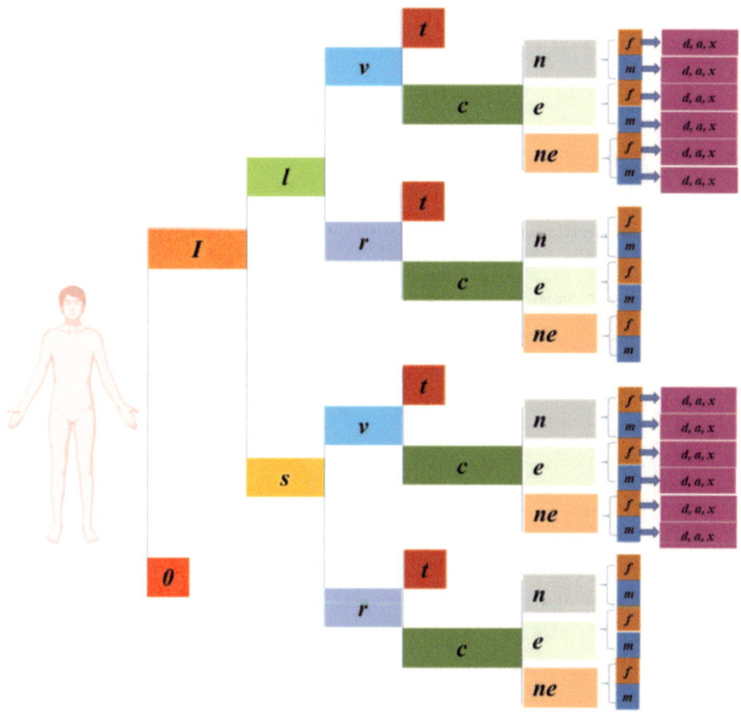

Figure 2.
Schematic representation of the different possible subsets of the contact and infection of human population with Taenia solium.

The set *I* includes at least 48 different subsets depending on whether the contact occurred a long (*l*) or short (*s*) time before sampling; the parasite was rejected (*r*) or it victoriously established in the host (*v*); the parasite is in the stage of a tapeworm (*t*) or as a cysticerci (*c*); if the cysticerci is located in the nervous system (*n*) or elsewhere (*e*) or in both (*ne*); if the cysticerci are few (*f*) or multiple (*m*); and if they are dead (*d*) or alive (*a*) or degenerating (*x*) (**Figure 2**).

The projection of positive serology upon the I set involve a number of immunological assumptions listed in **Table 1**.

Assuming the minimal, it may be concluded that:

1. Antibodies are to be found only in members of the *I* set in any of its subsets; and

2. Antigens are to be found only in members of the *I* subsets carrying live parasites at the time of sampling.

In consequence:

1. The finding of antibodies in an individual would be indicative of contact but would not establish the diagnosis of NC; and

2. The finding of antigen would establish the presence of a parasite in the form of cysticerci located either in the brain and/or elsewhere (i.e., skeletal muscle) or of an intestinal tapeworm.

If additional assumptions are added, then:

Minimal	1. Antigens used in the immunotest are specific of *T. solium* and present in all members of the species at all stages of development	
	2. There are no natural antibodies to the parasite.	
	3. There are no antiidiotipic antibodies simulating antigens.	
	4. All humans produce antibodies to at least a small and the same subset of the *T. solium* antigens in the immunotest.	
Additional	5. Antibodies and antigens tend to:	
		a. disappear with time after an unsuccessful attempt of the parasite to establish in the host,
		b. increase with the number of parasites established and
		c. concentrate in the compartment where the parasite is located.

Table 1.
Immunological assumptions involved upon positive serology within the I group (persons who has or had contact with Taenia solium*).*

3. Antibodies and antigens would be more likely (but not exclusively) to be found in all the *r* subsets of *I* that combine with *m* and *a* (that is, in all cysticercosis cases, acquired shortly or long before sampling, with many and live cysticerci located in the brain or elsewhere) and in tapeworm carriers. But more likely they would be found in the CSF in the neurocysticercosis (*n*) subsets combining with *m* and *a*, in the SERUM for the *e* (elsewhere cysticercosis) subsets also combining with *m* and *a*, and in the feces of *t* (carriers of live tapeworms). The precise magnitude of each likelihood is to be assessed in perhaps each endemic situation.

5. Clearing some discrepancy

From the above description of the variety in *T. solium* disease of humans and the usual and rather liberal assumptions about the quality of the immunological reactants and the nature of the immune response to this particular parasite many of the discrepancies in the performance of different immunotests in different trials may be explained. The most important being the variation in the composition of the set of control not-NC individuals (i.e., some containing more members of the *e* or *t* subsets of *I* would thwart specificity due to many false positive results) and/or in the control NC individuals (in which an undue number of the *d* subset would lower sensitivity). Likewise, the control NC individuals are frequently a mixed lot of NC patients, differing in time of evolution, number and location of cysticerci, form and time of medical and surgical treatment, general health and nutritional status, age, gender, race, etcetera, that can possibly affect their immune reactivity [39–46] (**Figure 3**).

The use of domestic and probably differently composed sets of presumed control *I* and *0* individuals and of NC and not-NC individuals accompanying each immunotest trial is widespread and thus suspect of being a major cause of incoherent results between trials.

Variation between different trials would also follow from differences in the probability distribution of immunologically positive and negative individuals in different situations of endemia (i.e., high and low endemia, urban and rural transmission) and in the simplification of the forms of disease by way of binomial variables (i.e., long or short time of exposure before sampling, single or multiple cysticerci,

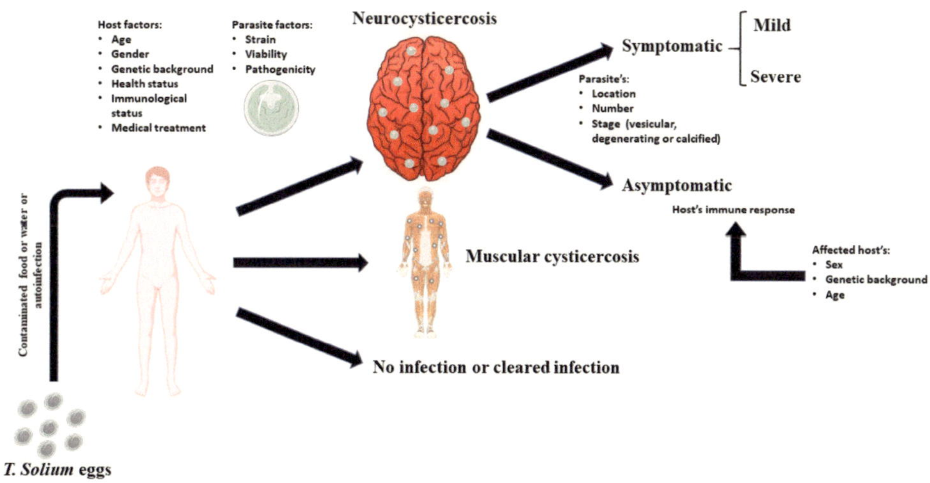

Figure 3.
Factors involved in neurocysticercosis. The development of neurocysticercosis depends on many factors from either the host or the parasite. The factors affecting the immune response of the host are particularly important for the immunodiagnosis of NC as they may affect the results between individuals.Differences in representativity of the whole of the parasite antigens and in cross-reactivity with other antigens in the geographic and endemic background, as well as differences in relative concentrations of reactants and conditions of reaction are additional suspect sources of variation.

dead or alive (not dying) when they are not really so (i.e., individual may be carrying 1, 2, ..., n cysticerci) and some are continuous (i.e., time of exposure before sampling) and even non-disjunctive (i.e. dead, degenerating and live cysticerci may coexist in an individual).

The selection of the *T. solium* antigens to be used as reactants in the immunotests also vary widely among the different immunotests and also within the same immunotest applied to different endemic conditions and geographic locations.

6. Immunological assumptions

Of all the immunological assumptions necessary to interpret the results of immuno tests in diagnosis of NC, the less tenable are those implying there are no cross-reactions with other parasites endemic in the area, that all humans react equally to infection and that the set of antigens selected for the immunotest are shared by all individual cysticerci and tapeworm in the species (**Figure 4**).

The question of antigen cross-reactivity is usually dealt-with by selection of the set of *T. solium* antigens most reactive with positive control samples (confirmed NC cases) and less reactive with negative control samples (presumably without NC), all gathered from donors residing in the endemic areas [47, 48]: a sensible procedure in principle but usually lacking in proof of the statistical representation of the population affected by the other pathogens and in the certainty of negative control samples with respect to clinically silent NC and cysticercosis located elsewhere. Failure to control antigen cross-reactivity results in false positive tests. That not all humans react equally to infection is an additional source of false negative immunotests. Heterogeneous immune response of humans to pathogens is well known in a number of infections, possibly all, and although not thoroughly explored in *T. solium* disease it follows from differences in levels of antibodies of control and problem samples as well as differences in the published images of WB [47–49]. Besides, NC cases donating samples to use as positive controls usually differ in some

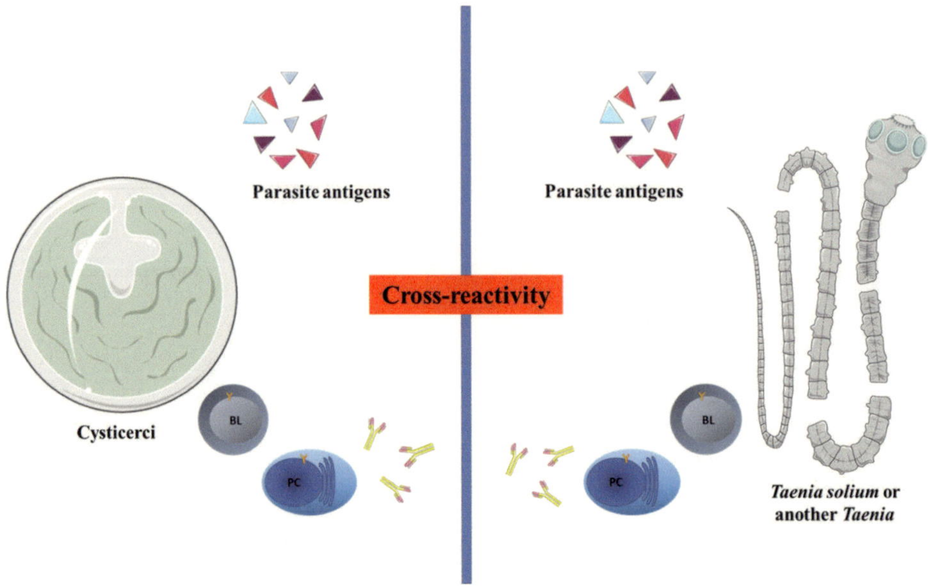

Figure 4.
Failure in immunodiagnosis. Cross-reactivity occurs due to some, but not all, of the secretion and excretion antigens of Taenia solium that are shared, not only during the different stages of its biological cycle, but also with some other endemic parasites (eg: Taenia saginata).

or various characteristics of the disease likely to be of immunological consequence (i.e., form and duration of treatment, natural history of the disease, site of residence, age [39], gender [40, 43–45, 50], race [28, 51–54]).

Thus, IDxNC is placed between the wall of false positives and the sword of false negatives and forced to negotiate selecting the antigen(s) most frequently found to react with control NC samples in order to decrease false positives but conceding some false negatives with the consequent loss in both sensitivity and specificity scores.

The antigen repertoire of *T. solium* is known to be numerous and varied [47, 48, 55, 56] but the distribution of the antigens in the members of the species, in the different developmental stages of the parasite and in different geographic locations is perhaps the most neglected possibly crucial need of information for the design of successful immunodiagnosis of *T. solium* disease.

7. Proposals for improvement

1. *T solium* disease is too serious a human problem to make of it an arena of scientific and technological individualistic rivalry. Cooperation is necessary to concert a worldwide effort to design an exacting research plan concordant with the complexities of *T. solium* disease and to develop and test in the short term a minimal number of options from which to select the most proficient IDxNC possible to be put to immediate production and general use while further research for improvement continues.

2. There is no hope for immunodiagnosis of *T. solium* disease without clearing the problem of antigen cross-reactivity and species representation. Purification of antigen(s) or epitopes critically certified to be exclusive of *T. solium* and present in all members of a representative sample of parasite specimens of an endemic site is mandatory. Although some likely candidates have been

proposed [55, 57, 58] they are lacking in satisfactorily meeting with either one or both of these conditions. A way of avoiding the high costs and demanding technical skills involved in the purification of natural antigens is the use of those present in phage display peptide libraries [59–61]. Antigens present in only *T. solium* but not in all specimens of the species would constitute the candidate antigen preparation (CAP).

3. It is also necessary to study and characterize the presumed wide spectrum of humans' antibody production in *T solium* disease in order to calibrate the candidate antigen preparation that would include all infected individuals. WBs using CAP in reaction with representative samples of all subsets of I, if possible, or of *n* and *e* at least, would provide the images necessary to construct all immunological profiles of the infected individuals. Computer assisted image analysis of WB and cluster analysis could address this problem. The set of CAP that reacts with all or most infected individuals would constitute the definitive antigen preparation (DAP).

4. Rather than attempting to develop ways to distinguish each of the different subsets of *T. solium* disease, efforts in immunodiagnosis could focus in improving diagnosis of NC (to include all subsets with *n* and *ne* to the exclusion of all other subsets of *I* as *t* and *e*), whilst for prevalence of *T. solium* disease, in whatever its form, it should only clearly distinguish members of the *I* set from those of *0*.

   Three are the classes of *T. solium* disease that matter the most and perhaps require different strategies: the contact case (members of the *I* set), the NC case (all *n* and *ne* subsets) and the tapeworm carrier (*t* subset). For this purpose, it is indispensable to construct representative and certified negative and positive control panels of the samples CSF, serum and feces from each geographic area upon their reaction with DAP. Certification of the members of the *e* subset and *0* set is complicated by its need of whole-body scans in search of cysticerci located elsewhere of CNS. Additional negative control samples from a culturally and historically certified community or geographic area to be rid of *T. solium* disease and low in infectious disease in general would be useful to estimate blank readings of immunotesting with DAP.

5. Once the problem of antigen specificity and representation is solved there should be no major problem to IDxNC in the CSF of a symptomatic neurological patient nor of an intestinal tapeworm in the feces, preferably by antigen detection (this, to distinguish cysticercosis located elsewhere and live from dead cysticerci in the CNS because antibodies could persist after death of the parasite for unknown periods of time).

6. But there would remain serious problems to tackle for serology, the most accessible sample useful for detection of early nonsymptomatic NC cases in the general population and for epidemiological studies of *T. solium* disease prevalence. The major problem for serology in unambiguously detecting asymptomatic NC cases is the potential location elsewhere of the parasite (all *e* subsets and the *t* subset) that produces false positive results, and the low reactivity of patients with few or calcified cysticerci (*f* and *d* subsets) that produces false negative results. Adding to positive serology a marker of CNS damage [62, 63] as a sign of CNS involvement could help in discriminating NC from other forms of *T. solium* disease.

Acknowledgements

This work was supported by Project Grants IN-209719 from Programa de Apoyo a Proyectos de Innovación Tecnológica (PAPIIT), Dirección General de Asuntos del Personal Académico (DGAPA), Universidad Nacional Autónoma de México (UNAM) and grant FC 2016-2125 from Fronteras en la Ciencia, Consejo Nacional de Ciencia y Tecnología (CONACYT), both granted to Jorge Morales-Montor. Project IA- 202919 from Programa de Apoyo a Proyectos de Investigación e Innovación Tecnológica (PAPIIT), Dirección General de Asuntos del Personal Académico (DGAPA), Universidad Nacional Autónoma de México (UNAM) to Karen Elizabeth Nava-Castro. Also project IA- 206220 from Programa de Apoyo a Proyectos de Investigación e Innovación Tecnológica (PAPIIT), Dirección General de Asuntos del Personal Académico (DGAPA), Universidad Nacional Autónoma de México (UNAM) to Víctor Hugo Del Río Araiza.

Conflict of interest

The authors declare no conflict of interest.

Author details

Marcela Esquivel-Velázquez[1], Carlos Larralde[1†], Pedro Ostoa-Saloma[1], Víctor Hugo Del Río Araiza[2] and Jorge Morales-Montor[1*]

1 Departamento de Inmunología, Instituto de Investigaciones Biomédicas, Universidad Nacional Autónoma de México (UNAM), Ciudad de México, Mexico

2 Departamento de Parasitología, Facultad de Medicina Veterinaria y Zootecnia, Universidad Nacional Autónoma de México (UNAM), Ciudad de México, Mexico

*Address all correspondence to: jmontor66@biomedicas.unam.mx

† Passed away

References

[1] F.W.H. Assembly, WORLD HEALTH ORGANIZATION FIFTY-FIFTH WORLD HEALTH ASSEMBLY A55/23 Provisional agenda item Control of neurocysticercosis Report by the Secretariat BACKGROUND, (2002).

[2] R.H.S. Peralta, A.J. Vaz, A. Pardini, H.W. Macedo, L.R. Machado, S.G. De Simone, J.M. Peralta, Evaluation of an antigen from Taenia crassiceps cysticercus for the serodiagnosis of neurocysticercosis, Acta Trop. 83 (2002) 159-168. https://doi.org/10.1016/S0001-706X(02)00092-X.

[3] V. Rajshekhar, G.G. Chacko, R.P. Haran, M.J. Chandy, S.M. Chandi, Clinicoradiological and pathological correlations in patients with solitary cysticercus granuloma and epilepsy: Focus on presence of the parasite and oedema formation, J. Neurol. Neurosurg. Psychiatry. 59 (1995) 284-286. https://doi.org/10.1136/jnnp.59.3.284.

[4] J. Sotelo, A. Flisser, Neuro cysticercosis. Practical treatment guidelines, CNS Drugs. 7 (1997) 17-25. https://doi.org/10.2165/00 23210-199707010-00003.

[5] A. Fleury, J. Moreno García, P. Valdez Aguerrebere, M. de Sayve Durán, P. Becerril Rodríguez, C. Larralde, E. Sciutto, Neurocysticercosis, a Persisting Health Problem in Mexico, PLoS Negl. Trop. Dis. 4 (2010) e805. https://doi.org/10.1371/journal.pntd.0000805.

[6] A. Fleury, M. Hernández, G. Fragoso, R.M.E. Parkhouse, L.J.S. Harrison, E. Sciutto, Detection of secreted cysticercal antigen: A useful tool in the diagnosis of inflammatory neurocysticercosis, Trans. R. Soc. Trop. Med. Hyg. 97 (2003) 542-546. https://doi.org/10.1016/S0035-9203(03)80019-6.

[7] A. Fleury, A. Escobar, G. Fragoso, E. Sciutto, C. Larralde, Clinical heterogeneity of human neurocysticercosis results from complex interactions among parasite, host and environmental factors, Trans. R. Soc. Trop. Med. Hyg. 104 (2010) 243-250. https://doi.org/10.1016/j.trstmh.2010.01.005.

[8] A. Flisser, T.W. Gyorkos, Contribution of immunodiagnostic tests to epidemiological/intervention studies of cysticercosis/taeniosis in México, Parasite Immunol. 29 (2007) 637-649. https://doi.org/10.1111/j.1365-3024.2007.00981.x.

[9] A. Carpio, Letter To The Editor: “Letter to the Editor,” J. Neurol. Sci. 161 (1998) 185-187. https://doi.org/10.1080/13518040701205365.

[10] E. Sarti, P.M. Schantz, A. Plancarte, M. Wilson, I.O. Gutierrez, J. Aguilera, J. Roberts, A. Flisser, Epidemiological investigation of Taenia solium taeniasis and cysticercosis in a rural village of Michoacan State, Mexico, Trans. R. Soc. Trop. Med. Hyg. 88 (1994) 49-52. https://doi.org/10.1016/0035-9203(94)90493-6.

[11] R.J. Bobes, M. Hernández, C. Márquez, G. Fragoso, E. García, R.M.E. Parkhouse, L.J.S. Harrison, E. Sciutto, A. Fleury, Subarachnoidal and intraventricular human neurocysticercosis: Application of an antigen detection assay for the diagnosis and follow-up, Trop. Med. Int. Heal. 11 (2006) 943-950. https://doi.org/10.1111/j.1365-3156.2006.01642.x.

[12] S.R.V. Atluri, P. Singhi, N. Khandelwal, N. Malla, Evaluation of excretory secretory and 10-30 kDa antigens of Taenia solium Cysticerci by EITB assay for the diagnosis of neurocysticercosis: Brief Definitive Report, Parasite Immunol. 31 (2009) 151-155. https://doi.org/10.1111/j.1365-3024.2008.01085.x.

[13] E.C. Bueno, M. Snege, A.J. Vaz, P.G. Leser, Serodiagnosis of human cysticercosis by using antigens from vesicular fluid of Taenia crassiceps cysticerci, Clin. Diagn. Lab. Immunol. 8 (2001) 1140-1144. https://doi.org/10.1128/CDLI.8.6.1140-1144.2001.

[14] S.R. V. Atluri, P. Singhi, N. Khandelwal, N. Malla, Neuro cysticercosis immunodiagnosis using Taenia solium cysticerci crude soluble extract, excretory secretory and lower molecular mass antigens in serum and urine samples of Indian children, Acta Trop. 110 (2009) 22-27. https://doi.org/10.1016/j.actatropica.2008.12.004.

[15] N. Malla, R. Kaur, N.K. Ganguly, I.M.S. Sawhney, R.C. Mahajan, Utility of specific IgG4 response in saliva and serum samples for the diagnosis and follow up of human neurocysticercosis., Nepal Med. Coll. J. 7 (2005) 1-9. https://europepmc.org/article/med/16295711 (accessed April 5, 2021).

[16] G. J.S., K. S., B. G., N.K. Ganguly, R.C. Mahajan, N. Malla, Kinetics of humoral & cellular immune responses in experimental cysticercosis in pigs infected with Taenia solium, Indian J Med Res. 111 (2000) 43-49. http://dx.doi.org/10.1016/j.jaci.2012.05.050.

[17] M. Maass, E. Delgado, J. Knobloch, Isolation of an immunodiagnostic Taenia solium coproantigen, Trop. Med. Parasitol. 43 (1992) 201-202. https://pubmed.ncbi.nlm.nih.gov/1470844/ (accessed April 5, 2021).

[18] M.-C. Guezala, S. Rodriguez, H. Zamora, H.H. Garcia, A.E. Gonzalez, A. Tembo, J.C. Allan, P.S. Craig, Development of a Species-Specific Coproantigen ELISA for Human Taenia solium Taeniasis, 2009.

[19] E.C. Bueno, A.J. Vaz, L. Dos Ramos Machado, J.A. Livramento, S.R. Mielle, Specific Taenia crassiceps and Taenia solium antigenic peptides for neurocysticercosis immunodiagnosis using serum samples, J. Clin. Microbiol. 38 (2000) 146-151. https://doi.org/10.1128/JCM.38.1.146-151.2000.

[20] J. Mandal, P.D. Singhi, N. Khandelwal, N. Malla, Evaluation of ELISA and dot blots for the serodiagnosis of neurocysticercosis, in children found to have single or multiple enhancing lesions in computerized tomographic scans of the brain, Ann. Trop. Med. Parasitol. 100 (2006) 39-48. https://doi.org/10.1179/136485906X78445.

[21] G.C. Arruda, A.D.T. Da Silva, E.M.A.B. Quagliato, M.A. Maretti, C.L. Rossi, Evaluation of Taenia solium and Taenia crassiceps cysticercal antigens for the serodiagnosis of neurocysticercosis, Trop. Med. Int. Heal. 10 (2005) 1005-1012. https://doi.org/10.1111/j.1365-3156.2005.01480.x.

[22] H.B. Oliveira, G.A. MacHado, M.D.R.F. Gonçalves-Pires, L.P. Moura, J.M. Costa-Cruz, Saline extract of Taenia saginata metacestodes as an alternative antigen for the immunodiagnosis of neurocysticercosis in human cerebrospinal fluid, Parasitol. Res. 105 (2009) 169-174. https://doi.org/10.1007/s00436-009-1379-z.

[23] V. Prabhakaran, V. Rajshekhar, K.D. Murrell, A. Oommen, Taenia solium metacestode glycoproteins as diagnostic antigens for solitary cysticercus granuloma in Indian patients, Trans. R. Soc. Trop. Med. Hyg. 98 (2004) 478-484. https://doi.org/10.1016/j.trstmh.2003.12.006.

[24] H.H. Garcia, R.M.E. Parkhouse, R.H. Gilman, T. Montenegro, T. Bernal, S.M. Martinez, A.E. Gonzalez, V.C.W. Tsang, L.J.S. Harrison, Serum antigen detection in the diagnosis, treatment, and follow-up of neurocysticercosis patients, Trans. R. Soc. Trop. Med. Hyg. 94 (2000) 673-676. https://doi.org/10.1016/S0035-9203(00)90228-1.

[25] J.A. Lopez, E. Garcia, I.M. Cortes, J. Sotelo, P. Tato, J.L. Molinari, Neurocysticercosis: Relationship between the developmental stage of metacestode present and the titre of specific IgG in the cerebrospinal fluid, Ann. Trop. Med. Parasitol. 98 (2004) 569-579. https://doi.org/10.1179/000349804225021424.

[26] J.L. Molinari, E. García-Mendoza, Y. De la Garza, J.A. Ramírez, J. Sotelo, P. Tato, Discrimination between active and inactive neurocysticercosis by metacestode excretory/secretory antigens of Taenia solium in an enzyme-linked immunosorbent assay, Am. J. Trop. Med. Hyg. 66 (2002) 777-781. https://doi.org/10.4269/ajtmh.2002.66.777.

[27] P.S. Sahu, S.C. Parija, S.K. Narayan, D. Kumar, Evaluation of an IgG-ELISA strategy using Taenia solium metacestode somatic and excretory-secretory antigens for diagnosis of neurocysticercosis revealing biological stage of the larvae, Acta Trop. 110 (2009) 38-45. https://doi.org/10.1016/j.actatropica.2009.01.002.

[28] V. Prabhakaran, V. Rajshekhar, K.D. Murrell, A. Oommen, Conformation-sensitive immunoassays improve the serodiagnosis of solitary cysticercus granuloma in Indian patients, Trans. R. Soc. Trop. Med. Hyg. 101 (2007) 570-577. https://doi.org/10.1016/j.trstmh.2006.10.001.

[29] H.H. Garcia, O.H. Del Brutto, Neurocysticercosis: Updated concepts about an old disease, Lancet Neurol. 4 (2005) 653-661. https://doi.org/10.1016/S1474-4422(05)70194-0.

[30] L. Salim, A. Ang, S. Handali, V.C.W. Tsang, Seroepidemiologic survey of cysticercosis-taeniasis in four central highland districts of papua, indonesia, Am. J. Trop. Med. Hyg. 80 (2009) 384-388. https://doi.org/10.4269/ajtmh.2009.80.384.

[31] R.M. Greene, K. Hancock, P.P. Wilkins, V.C.W. Tsang, TAENIA SOLIUM: MOLECULAR CLONING AND SEROLOGIC EVALUATION OF 14- AND 18-KDA RELATED, DIAGNOSTIC ANTIGENS, Https://Doi.Org/10.1645/0022-3395(2000)086[1001:TSMCAS]2.0.CO;2. 86 (2000) 1001-1007. https://doi.org/10.1645/0022-3395(2000)086[1001,TSMCAS]2.0.CO;2.

[32] M. Hernández, C. Beltrán, E. García, G. Fragoso, G. Gevorkian, A. Fleury, M. Parkhouse, L. Harrison, J. Sotelo, E. Sciutto, Cysticercosis: Towards the design of a diagnostic kit based on synthetic peptides, Immunol. Lett. 71 (2000) 13-17. https://doi.org/10.1016/S0165-2478(99)00166-2.

[33] C.M. Scheel, A. Khan, K. Hancock, H.H. Garcia, A.E. Gonzalez, R.H. Gilman, V.C.W. Tsang, H. Mayta, M.T. Lopez, M. Silva, S. Rodriguez, J. Noh, Serodiagnosis of neurocysticercosis using synthetic 8-KD proteins: Comparison of assay formats, Am. J. Trop. Med. Hyg. 73 (2005) 771-776. https://doi.org/10.4269/ajtmh.2005.73.771.

[34] M.M.I. Ishida, R.H.S. Peralta, J.A. Livramento, S. Hoshino-Shimizu, J.M. Peralta, A.J. Vaz, Serodiagnosis of neurocysticercosis in patients with epileptic seizure using ELISA and immunoblot assay, Rev. Inst. Med. Trop. Sao Paulo. 48 (2006) 343-346. https://doi.org/10.1590/S0036-46652006000600008.

[35] H.B. Oliveira, G.A. Machado, D.D. Cabral, J.M. Costa-Cruz, Application of Taenia saginata metacestodes as an alternative antigen for the serological diagnosis of human neurocysticercosis, Parasitol. Res. 101 (2007) 1007-1013. https://doi.org/10.1007/s00436-007-0578-8.

[36] N. Shukla, N. Husain, Jyotsna, S. Gupta, M. Husain, Comparisons

between scolex and membrane antigens of Cysticercus fasciolaris and Cysticercus cellulosae larvae for immunodiagnosis of neurocysticercosis, J. Microbiol. Immunol. Infect. 41 (2008) 519-524. https://europepmc.org/article/med/19255697 (accessed April 5, 2021).

[37] M. Ramos Kuri, J. Sotelo, R.M. Montoya, A. Padilla, T. Govezensky, M.L. Diaz, E. Sciutto, C. Larralde, Immunodiagnosis of Neurocysticercosis: Disappointing Performance of Serology (Enzyme-Linked Immunosorbent Assay) in an Unbiased Sample of Neurological Patients, Arch. Neurol. 49 (1992) 633-636. https://doi.org/10.1001/archneur.1992.00530300069012.

[38] S.J. Furrows, J. McCroddan, W.J. Bligh, P. Chiodini, Lack of specificity of a single positive 50-kDa band in the electroimmunotransfer blot (EITB) assay for cysticercosis, Clin. Microbiol. Infect. 12 (2006) 459-462. https://doi.org/10.1111/j.1469-0691.2006.01381.x.

[39] A. Fleury, A. Dessein, P.M. Preux, M. Dumas, G. Tapia, C. Larralde, E. Sciutto, Symptomatic human neurocysticercosis: Age, sex and exposure factors relating with disease heterogeneity, J. Neurol. 251 (2004) 830-837. https://doi.org/10.1007/s00415-004-0437-9.

[40] J. Morales-Montor, A. Chavarria, M.A. De León, L.I. Del Castillo, E.G. Escobedo, E.N. Sánchez, J.A. Vargas, M. Hernández-Flores, T. Romo-González, C. Larralde, HOST GENDER IN PARASITIC INFECTIONS OF MAMMALS: AN EVALUATION OF THE FEMALE HOST SUPREMACY PARADIGM, J. Parasitol. 90 (2004) 531-546. https://doi.org/10.1645/GE-113R3.

[41] J. Morales-Montor, S. Baig, C. Hallal-Calleros, R.T. Damian, Taenia crassiceps: Androgen reconstitution of the host leads to protection during cysticercosis, Exp. Parasitol. 100 (2002) 209-216. https://doi.org/10.1016/S0014-4894(02)00028-0.

[42] I. Marriott, Y.M. Huet-Hudson, Sexual dimorphism in innate immune responses to infectious organisms, Immunol. Res. 34 (2006) 177-192. https://doi.org/10.1385/IR:34:3:177.

[43] A. Chavarría, A. Fleury, E. García, C. Márquez, G. Fragoso, E. Sciutto, Relationship between the clinical heterogeneity of neurocysticercosis and the immune-inflammatory profiles, Clin. Immunol. 116 (2005) 271-278. https://doi.org/10.1016/j.clim.2005.04.008.

[44] O.H. Del Brutto, E. García, O. Talámas, J. Sotelo, Sex-Related Severity of Inflammation in Parenchymal Brain Cysticercosis, Arch. Intern. Med. 148 (1988) 544-546. https://doi.org/10.1001/archinte.1988.00380 030050011.

[45] A. Fleury, T. Gomez, I. Alvarez, D. Meza, M. Huerta, A. Chavarria, R.A. Carrillo Mezo, C. Lloyd, A. Dessein, P.M. Preux, M. Dumas, C. Larralde, E. Sciutto, G. Fragoso, High prevalence of calcified silent neurocysticercosis in a rural village of Mexico, Neuroepidemiology. 22 (2003) 139-145. https://doi.org/10.1159/000068748.

[46] S. Khurana, A. Aggarwal, N. Malla, Prevalence of anti-cysticercus antibodies in slum, rural and urban populations in and around Union territory, Chandigarh., Indian J Pathol Microbiol . 49 (2006) 51-53.

[47] V.C.W. Tsang, J.A. Brand, A.E. Boyer, An Enzyme-Linked Immunoelectrotransfer Blot Assay and Glycoprotein Antigens for Diagnosing Human Cysticercosis (Taenia solium), J. Infect. Dis. 159 (1989) 50-59. https://doi.org/10.1093/infdis/159.1.50.

[48] C. Larralde, R.M. Montoya, E. Sciutto, M.L. Diaz, T. Govezensky, E.

Coltorti, Deciphering western blots of tapeworm antigens (Taenia solium, Echinococcus granulosus, and Taenia crassiceps) reacting with sera from neurocysticercosis and hydatid disease patients, Am. J. Trop. Med. Hyg. 40 (1989) 282-290. https://doi.org/10.4269/ajtmh.1989.40.282.

[49] C. Larralde, A. Padilla, M. Hernández, T. Govezensky, E. Sciutto, G. Gutiérrez, R. Tapia-Conyer, B. Salvatierra, J. Sepúlveda, [Seroepidemiology of cysticercosis in Mexico]., Salud Publica Mex. 34 (1992) 197-210. http://www.ncbi.nlm.nih.gov/pubmed/1631733.

[50] D. Verthelyi, Sex hormones as immunomodulators in health and disease, Int. Immunopharmacol. 1 (2001) 983-993. https://doi.org/10.1016/S1567-5769(01)00044-3.

[51] G. Singh, Neurocysticercosos in South-Central America and the Indian subcontinent. A comparative evaluation., Arq. Neuropsiquiatr. 55 (1997) 349-356. https://doi.org/10.1590/S0004-282X1997000300001.

[52] M. Tibayrenc, Human Genetic Diversity and the Epidemiology of Parasitic and Other Transmissible Diseases, Adv. Parasitol. 64 (2007) 377-462. https://doi.org/10.1016/S0065-308X(06)64004-9.

[53] S.C. Shafir, F.J. Sorvillo, L. Smith, Current issues and considerations regarding Trichomoniasis and human immunodeficiency virus in African-Americans, Clin. Microbiol. Rev. 22 (2009) 37-45. https://doi.org/10.1128/CMR.00002-08.

[54] C. Alves, T. Souza, I. Meyer, M.B.P. Toralles, C. Brites, Immunogenetics and infectious diseases: Special reference to the mayor histocompatibility complex, Brazilian J. Infect. Dis. 10 (2006) 122-131. https://doi.org/10.1590/S1413-86702006000200010.

[55] E. Garcia, G. Ordonez, J. Sotelo, Antigens from Taenia crassiceps cysticerci used in complement fixation, enzyme-linked immunosorbent assay, and Western blot (immunoblot) for diagnosis of neurocysticercosis, J. Clin. Microbiol. 33 (1995) 3324-3325. https://doi.org/10.1128/jcm.33.12.3324-3325.1995.

[56] A.J. Vaz, C.M. Nunes, R.M.F. Piazza, J.A. Livramento, M. V. Da Silva, P.M. Nakamura, A.W. Ferreira, Immunoblot with cerebrospinal fluid from patients with neurocysticercosis using antigen from cysticerci of Taenia solium and Taenia crassiceps, Am. J. Trop. Med. Hyg. 57 (1997) 354-357. https://doi.org/10.4269/ajtmh.1997.57.354.

[57] E.G. Lee, Y.A. Bae, S.H. Kim, S.P. Díaz-Camacho, Y. Nawa, Y. Kong, Serodiagnostic reliability of single-step enriched low-molecular weight proteins of Taenia solium metacestode of American and Asian isolates, Trans. R. Soc. Trop. Med. Hyg. 104 (2010) 676-683. https://doi.org/10.1016/j.trstmh.2010.07.011.

[58] S. Handali, M. Klarman, A.N. Gaspard, J. Noh, Y.M. Lee, S. Rodriguez, A.E. Gonzalez, H.H. Garcia, R.H. Gilman, V.C.W. Tsang, P.P. Wilkins, Multiantigen print immunoassay for comparison of diagnostic antigens for Taenia solium cysticercosis and taeniasis, Clin. Vaccine Immunol. 17 (2010) 68-72. https://doi.org/10.1128/CVI.00339-09.

[59] A. Fleury, C. Beltran, E. Ferrer, T. Garate, L.J.S. Harrison, R.M.E. Parkhouse, E. Garcia, G. Fragoso, J. Costa-Cruz, G. Biondi, S. Agapejev, E. Sciutto, Application of synthetic peptides to the diagnosis of neurocysticercosis, Trop. Med. Int. Heal. 8 (2003) 1124-1130. https://doi.org/10.1046/j.1360-2276.2003.01132.x.

[60] V. da Silva Ribeiro, M.N. Manhani, R. Cardoso, C.U. Vieira, L.R. Goulart,

J.M. Costa-Cruz, Selection of high affinity peptide ligands for detection of circulating antibodies in neurocysticercosis, Immunol. Lett. 129 (2010) 94-99. https://doi.org/10.1016/j.imlet.2010.01.008.

[61] K. Gazarian, M. Rowley, T. Gazarian, J. Sotelo, E. Mendoza, R. Hernandez, Post-Panning Computer-Aided Analysis of Phagotope Collections Selected with Neurocysticercosis Patient Polyclonal Antibodies Separation of Disease-Relevant and Irrelevant Peptide Sequences, Comb. Chem. High Throughput Screen. 4 (2012) 221-235. https://doi.org/10.2174/13862070 13331156.

[62] T. Schmitz, U. Felderhoff-Mueser, M. Sifringer, F. Groenendaal, S. Kampmann, A. Heep, Expression of soluble Fas in the cerebrospinal fluid of preterm infants with posthemorrhagic hydrocephalus and cystic white matter damage, J. Perinat. Med. 39 (2011) 83-88. https://doi.org/10.1515/JPM.2010.125.

[63] R.L. Hayes, G. Robinson, U. Muller, K.K.W. Wang, Translation of neurological biomarkers to clinically relevant platforms, Methods Mol. Biol. 566 (2009) 303-313. https://doi.org/10.1007/978-1-59745-562-6_20.

Section 3

New Leading Compounds as Possible Drug Targets in Cysticercosis

Chapter 5

Taenia solium microRNAs: Potential Biomarkers and Drug Targets in Neurocysticercosis

Matías Gastón Pérez

Abstract

MicroRNAs (miRNAs) found in animals, plants, and some viruses belongs to the heterogeneous class of non-coding RNAs (ncRNAs), which posttranscriptional regulates gene expression. They are linked to various cellular activities such as cell growth, differentiation, development and apoptosis. Also, they have been involved in cancer, metabolic diseases, viral infections and clinical trials targeting miRNAs has shown promising results. This chapter provides an overview on *Taenia solium* and *Taenia crassiceps* miRNAs, their possible biological functions, their role in host–parasite communication and their potential role as biomarkers and drug targets.

Keywords: miRNAs, small noncoding RNAs, neurocysticercosis, biomarkers, drug target

1. Introduction

1.1 Overview of miRNAs: definition, biogenesis, and functions

MicroRNAs (miRNAs) are a major class of small noncoding RNAs (ncRNAs) found in animals, plants, and some viruses, which negatively regulate gene expression at the messenger RNA (mRNA) level [1]. The first known miRNA (lin-4) was found in the free-living nematode *Caenorhabditis elegans* [2]. Seven years later let-7 was identified, and together with lin-4 were found to regulate developmental timing of *C. elegans* larvae [3]. By definition, miRNAs are small RNA molecules incapable of encoding proteins, but possessing important structural, catalytic, and regulatory functions comprise one of the more abundant classes of gene regulatory molecules in multicellular organisms and likely influence the output of many protein-coding genes. According to the latest miRBase release (v22.1, October 2018, http://www.mirbase.org/), there are miRNAs from 271 species, expressing 38589 mature miRNAs.

It is well established that miRNA biogenesis is a complex process classified into canonical and non-canonical pathways. The canonical biogenesis is the dominant pathway by which miRNAs are processed [4]. This pathway includes three main steps: (i) In the nucleus, miRNA genes are transcript by RNA polymerase II as part of much longer RNAs called pri-miRNAs which contain one or a few stem-loop structures composed of approximately 70 nucleotides each (**Figure 1**). Sometimes miRNAs are transcribed as one long transcript called clusters, which may have similar seed regions, and in which case they are considered a family [5]. About half of all currently identified miRNAs are intragenic and processed

IntechOpen

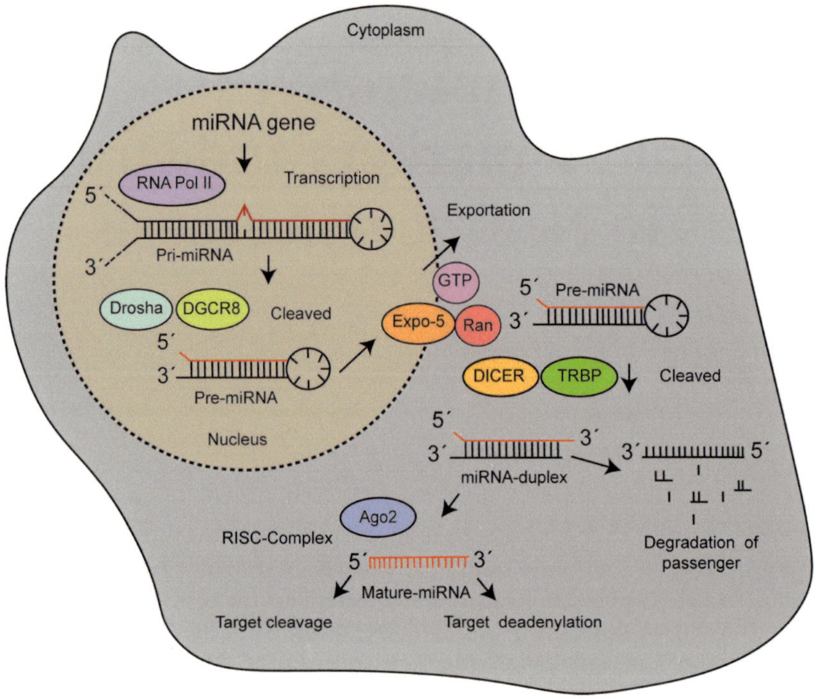

Figure 1.
Canonical microRNA biogenesis and mechanism of action. The biogenesis begins with the generation of the pri-miRNA transcript by RNA polymerase II in the nucleus. The microprocessor complex, composed of Drosha and DiGeorge syndrome critical region 8 (DGCR8), cleaves the pri-miRNA to produce the precursor-miRNA (pre-miRNA). After translocation into the cytoplasm by exportin 5, pre-miRNAs are processed by Dicer to form the mature miRNA/miRNA duplex. Following processing, miRNAs are assembled into the RISC complex. Only one strand of the duplex is stably associated with the RISC complex. The mature miRNA directs repression of mRNA containing complementary miRNA binding sites within the 3'UTR.*

mostly from introns and relatively few exons of protein coding genes, while the remaining are intergenic, transcribed independently of a host gene and regulated by their own promoters [6] (ii) Then, the microprocessor complex, consisting of an RNA binding protein DiGeorge Syndrome Critical Region 8 (DGCR8) and a ribonuclease III enzyme, Drosha trims the pri-miRNA to liberate a pre-miRNA hairpin which is actively transported to the cytoplasm by 5 (XPO5)/RanGTP complex (**Figure 1**) (iii) Its final maturation is processed in the cytoplasm where Dicer RNase III endonuclease cleaves the pre-miRNA into a single-stranded mature miRNA, removing the terminal loop (**Figure 1**) [4]. The directionality of the miRNA strand determines the name of the mature miRNA form [5]. Subsequently, with assistance from chaperone proteins (HSC70/HSP90) the mature miRNA is loaded into proteins of the Argonaute (Ago) family and assembles the RNA induced silencing complex (RISC) together to exert its further physiological functions (**Figure 1**). We defined the unloaded strand as passenger or star strand. The start strand that contains no mismatches are cleaved by AGO2 and degraded (**Figure 1**). Also, miRNA duplexes with central mismatches or non-AGO2 loaded miRNA are unwound and degraded. After being incorporated into the RISC, the mature miRNA induces posttranscriptional gene silencing by tethering RISC to be partially complementary to the target mRNA predominantly found within the 3′-untranslated regions (UTR). Targeting can also be facilitated by additional sequence elements, such as an unpaired Adenosine in the mRNA target sequence, corresponding to the nucleotide 1 in 5′ end of the mature miRNA. On the other hand, non-canonical miRNA biogenesis pathways are grouped into

Drosha/DGCR8-independent and Dicer-independent pathways. In general, these pathways make use of different combinations of the proteins involved in the canonical pathway, mainly Drosha, Dicer, exportin 5, and AGO2 [4].

It has been estimated that miRNAs regulate the expression of approximately one-third of the protein-coding genes [1]. Each miRNA can have many target mRNAs and a single mRNA can be regulated by multiple miRNAs [7]. Given this vast majority of mRNA targets regulated by miRNAs, aberrant miRNA expression profoundly influences a wide variety of cell regulation pathways important to cell proliferation, apoptosis, and stress responses.

Single miRNA gene can generate multiple miRNA isoforms (isomiRs). For example, the inconsistent choice of the strand loaded into AGO can generate two different functional miRNAs from both strands of the pre-miRNA duplex [8]. Imprecise cleavage of pri-miRNA by Drosha or pre-miRNA by Dicer can generate heterogeneous 5′ or 3′ ends. Another way to generate isomiRs is by RNA editing which may have a functional impact when the seed nucleotide is altered [4]. Exonuclease activity could remove nucleotides from miRNA 3′ end, and terminal nucleotide-transferase could add nucleotides to the miRNA 3′ end generating different isomiRs.

For almost a decade, some of the miRNA genes have been categorized into different groups, named miRNA families, based on the mature miRNA sequence and/or structure of pre-miRNAs [9]. Thus, means that microRNAs are grouped into families based on their targeting properties, which depend primarily on the identity of their extended seed region (miRNA nucleotides 2–8) [10]. Interestingly, it has been observed that miRNA genes in the same miRNA family are non-randomly co-localized and well organized around genes involved in infectious, immune system, sensory system and neurodegenerative diseases, development and cancer [11]. As with paralogous proteins, members of the same seed families often have at least partially redundant functions, with severe loss-of-function phenotypes apparent only after multiple family members are disrupted [12].

Biological functions of individual miRNAs have been extensively explored and have revealed the important role of miRNAs in many biological functions such as developmental timings, cell differentiation, embryogenesis, metabolism, organogenesis, and apoptosis [13]. Thus, miRNAs have been introduced as therapeutics or as targets of therapeutics for the treatment of disease [14]. Also, the existence of extracellular miRNAs has been widely reported these molecules as potential biomarkers for a variety of diseases. At present, miRNAs-mediated therapies for treatment of cancer and chronic hepatitis C virus (HCV) infection have shown promising results in human Phase I clinical trial [15].

2. miRNAs in *Taenia solium* and *Taenia crassiceps*

The presence of homologs to Drosha, Dicer, and Pasha (as identified in the *T. solium* Genome Project) [16] and the differences in miRNAs profiles between the *Taenia solium* cysticerci and adults suggest that the process for the synthesis of miRNAs is similar to that described for mammals. Identification and sequencing of miRNAs have been largely facilitated by the newly available high-throughput tools that have generated a growing set of miRNA sequences from parasites. Our group report for the first time the high confidence miRNA repertoire from *T. crassiceps* and *T. solium* and show that miRNAs account for most small RNA expression in *T. crassiceps* cysticerci by small RNA-seq experiments [17]. Since our miRNA identification strategy required the matching of *T. crassiceps* small RNA sequences to the *T. solium* genome, the identified miRNAs are considered common to both species, as was previously considered for other helminth parasites [18, 19]. The percentage of miRNAs in *T. crassiceps* cysticerci reaches 83% of the total small RNA expression, suggesting important functions of this type of RNA in the biology of taenias [17]. Also, miRNAs were identified and validated by northern blot experiments [17]. This validation is especially important in the case that genomic data from other species is used. Additionally, we experimentally detected pre-miRNAs for the first time in cestodes adding confidence to the miRNA identification procedure performed [17]. The *T. solium* and *T. crassiceps* miRNA catalog includes 41 conserved miRNAs grouped into 30 families [17]. The number of conserved miRNA families is similar to that of *Echinococcus canadensis* [20] and *Mesocestoides vogae* (syn: *M. corti*) [21] (28 conserved miRNA families), providing further evidence for the loss of conserved miRNA families in cestodes [22]. In *T. solium* genome it was reported two miRNA precursors (pre-mir-new-1a and pre-mir-new-1b) arranged in a cluster [17] that were only reported before for the *Echinococcus granulosus* s. s. G1 genotype [23]. The first of these precursors shows expression from both arms in *T. crassiceps*, unlike the *E. granulosus* s. s. G1 genotype that only expressed the 3p arm [17]. Differences in the genome organization of miRNA precursors among cestodes was reported. For example, the cluster miR-7b and miR-3479a found in *T. solium* are not clustered in *Echinococcus* or *M. vogae* [17]. The cluster miR-71/2c/2b, it was found only once in the genome of *T. solium*, as observed in other cestodes analyzed to date [20, 21, 24]. The presence of only one miR-71/miR-2 cluster seems to be a common feature of cestode genomes. The uneven expression found among miRNAs of this cluster was also observed in *Echinococcus* spp. [20, 24] and *M. vogae* [21]. Cluster miRNAs are evolutionally and functionally related and may co-regulate multiple biological processes. Additionally, cluster miRNAs have shown to evolve more rapidly than individual miRNAs [25]. Current evidence in humans suggests that, various genetic events (deletion, insertion, duplication and base substitution) within a cluster, followed by adaption and neofunctionalization, is the underlying mechanism responsible for the evolution of miRNA clusters [26]. To date, the importance of these differences in genomic arrangement of cestodes is unknown but could potentially influence the expression of the corresponding mature miRNAs.

The expression profile of *T. crassiceps* cysticerci showed that miRNA expression is highly biased to a few miRNAs: miR-10, let-7, miR-71, bantam and miR-61 [17]. These five miRNAs account for ~90% of miRNA expression [17]. These miRNAs and miR-4989 were also highly expresses in *Taenia solium* cysticerci [27]. Coincidentally, in other reports of small RNAs from cestodes that used the same methodology for miRNA discovery, miR-10, let-7, miR-71 and bantam were the most highly expressed, suggesting important functions in cestode biology [20, 21, 23, 24]. The repertoire of miRNAs in *T. solium* genome included protostomian miRNAs, such as miR-4989 and bantam that are absent in human host [17]. MiR-4989 is a divergent member of the miR-277 family. This protostomian-specific family is known to be involved in amino acid catabolism in *Drosophila*. Recently, miR-4989 was shown to be involved in development of juvenile worms in *S. mansoni*. In the *T. solium* genome miR-4989 target a Cationic amino acid transporter and a basic leucine zipper bZIP transcription factor without orthologs in any model species. Additionally, in the genome of *T. solium* and expressed in *T. crassiceps* cysticerci we found bilaterian miRNAs that are absent in human host, such as miR-71 or divergent from their host ortholog, such as let-7 [17].

The identification and characterization of miRNA targets is essential for understanding the function of these ncRNAs at molecular level. MiR-10 is the most expressed miRNA in *T. crassiceps* and *T. solium* cysticerci. This miRNA is highly conserved across metazoan organisms and is implicated in Hox gene regulation, embryonic development, and cancer [28–30]. Tow ANTP class homeobox genes were found among predicted miR-10 targets in *T. solium* genome [17] as in many others bilaterians [31]. Let-7, a conserved miRNA across evolution, was shown to regulate the developmental timing in *C. elegans* [32] and was shown to be a central regulator of mammalian glucose metabolism by targeting several genes of the insulin-PI3K-mTor pathway, including the insulin receptor [33]. MiR-9 is a deeply conserved miRNA across evolution known to be involved in neural development. One possible target for miR-9 is a Slit 2 protein, the ortholog of *C. elegans* slt-1 that is expressed in muscle cells and neurons and is involved in generation of neurons and axon guidance during embryonic and larval development. Also, a Carbonic anhydrase was reported as a putative target gene for miR-9, which is the ortholog of *C. elegans* cah-1 that is expressed in different neurons and head ganglion and is predicted to have a carbonate dehydratase activity. Other relevant target for miR-9 was Peregrin, the ortholog of *C. elegans* lin-49 that is involved in normal larval development. MiR-71 is bilaterian miRNA absent in vertebrates and involved in the promotion of longevity and neuronal asymmetry in *C. elegans,* is the miRNA with more targets predicted in the genome of *Taenia solium.* Some interesting targets are shown in **Table 1**.

Parasite miRNAs that are absent in the host, such as miR-71 or highly divergent (e.g let-7) from their host orthologs may be considered as selective therapeutic targets for treatment and control of helminth parasite infections. In addition, miR-71 is highly expressed in *T. solium* adults stage suggesting that it could be involved in important biological functions in the life cycle of *Taenia* genus. Nevertheless, the characterization of the physiological effects of the presence or absence for each identified miRNA needs more complex approaches in *T. solium*. In this respect, in vitro and in vivo optimization strategies for efficient and long-lasting loss-of-function, such miR-71 silencing reported in *E. multilocularis* [34] are still required for meaningful silencing studies in other metacestodes.

2.1 miRNAs and immune response

Helminth's parasites modulate immune responses in their host to prevent their elimination and establish chronic infections. Neurocysticercosis (NCC) implicates chronic parasitic disease with different variety of host and parasite interactions [35]. Clinical manifestations are mainly the result of inflammatory response to degeneration of parenchymal cysticercus [36].

Taenia solium cysticerci actively prevents this inflammatory response [37], which prolongs its survival in the host. The intensity of NCC symptoms depends primarily on the inflammatory response, which is associated with the Th1 response with high levels of TNF, IFN-γ, IL-17, and IL-23 whereas the Th2 response (anti-inflammatory response) is associated with asymptomatic NCC with high level of IL-10, IL- 4, IL5, and IL-13 [38]. In *T. crassiceps* model, the cysticercus growth is controlled by macrophages and the promoting of Th1 and Th2 responses. The production of inflammatory cytokines by macrophages and dendritic cells are blocked by excreted/secreted antigens (E-S antigens). Also, toll-like receptor (TLR) are blocked facilitating cysticercus growth [38]. The miRNA signature of T regulatory (Treg) cells has been characterized and among the miRNAs expressed are mir-21 and mir-31, which have opposing effects on the Treg TF FOXP3 [38]. Also, it was demonstrated that the E-S antigens of *T. crassiceps* cysticerci can modulate proinflammatory responses in macrophages by inducing regulatory posttranscriptional mechanisms, while E-S antigens reduced the production of inflammatory cytokines (IL-6, IL-12, and TNFα), they increased the release of IL-10 in LPS-induced bone marrow-derived macrophages [39]. microRNAs are a key component of macrophage posttranscriptional regulation [40] and it was shown that E-S antigens of *T. crassiceps* cysticerci induced upregulation of miR-125a-5p, miR-762, and miR-484, which are predicted to target canonical inflammatory molecules and pathways in LPS-induced bone marrow-derived macrophages.

Gene ID	Gene description	Molecular funtion (GO)	Other miRNAs
TsM_001055500	Zinc finger, type RING / FYVE / PHD	—	bantam; miR-4989
TsM_001107400	Ubiquitin carboxyl terminal hydrolase (inferred by orthology to a protein from *S. mansoni*)	Thiol-dependent ubiquitinyl hydrolase activity	miR-36a; miR-36b
TsM_000718200	Ceramide glucosyltransferase (inferred by orthology to a human protein)	Transferase activity, transfer of glycosyl groups	let-7
TsM_000983300	Casp, putative (inferred by orthology to a protein from S. mansoni)	—	miR-71
TsM_000787600	Protein kinase-like domain. Tyrosine-protein kinase, active site.	Protein kinase activity, protein serine / threonine kinase activity, ATP binding, phosphotransferase activity, alcohol group as acceptor	miR-9
TsM_000964500	IUAA Family Transporter	—	miR-10
TsM_000502500	Fibroblast growth factor receptor homolog 1 (inferred by orthology to a *D. melanogaster* protein)	Protein kinase activity, protein tyrosine kinase activity, ATP binding	miR-124a; miR-124b
TsM_000692000	Mitochondrial coenzyme transporter A SLC25A42 (inferred by orthology to a human protein)	—	miR-61

Table 1.
Interesting miR-71 targets in Taenia solium *genome.*

Taenia solium E-S antigens have been implicated in immune modulation and it is also known that the intimate association between host and parasite and the immune response is highly controlled at the post transcriptional level [41]. Target prediction of miR-10 and miR-125 found in *T. solium* cysticerci are potentially involved in macrophage IRF/STAT pathways, such as CD69 and TNF. Also, miR-9 was found to be related in the classical activation of macrophages [38]. Mir-10 and miR-125 were also implicated in expression of cytokine receptors, cell activation markers and cell adhesion molecules that activate macrophages to secrete TNF involved in IFN-signaling pathway. Furthermore, potential miR-10 targets such as IL12 and IL23, could interfere with the IL-12 family signaling pathway with a probably Tregs induction. In addition, let-7 showed predicted targets, such as IL10 that encodes cytokines involved in M2 polarization [42]. These suggest an important role in the polarization of macrophages. Macrophages in cysticercosis promote a transient Th1 protective response with classical activated macrophages that is changed by parasite products to a Th2 permissive response with alternatively activated macrophages [43].

Already knowing that the more abundant miRNAs (miR-10-5p, let-7-5p) putatively have target genes of immune response and that macrophages in murine cysticercosis promote Th1 or Th2 responses it was demonstrated that synthetic miR-10-5p and let-7-5p were internalized into the cytoplasm of murine peritoneal macrophages in vitro [27]. Interestingly, the down regulation of the expression of pro-inflammatory cytokines, such as Il6, Il1b, and TNF, IL-12, was reported when activated macrophages were incubated with IFN-γ and miR-10-5p or let-7-5p.

Moreover, in macrophages activated with IL-4 these miRNAs reduced the expression of cytokines involved in M2/Th2 differentiation. These results were important, because murine resistant to cysticercosis display high levels of TNF, IL-12, IL1-β, and NO during early infection (Th1 response), which is associated with the elimination of larvae [44]. On the other hand, high levels of pro-inflammatory cytokines (IL-6 and TNF) cause damage to the microglia promoting autoimmune and neurodegenerative diseases [45, 46]. This tissue damage is also observed in human NCC at the beginning of larvae degeneration and in pig NCC when they are treated with praziquantel [47]. In contrast, viable larvae are associated with a long initial asymptomatic phase that correlate with undetectable inflammation in the SNC, presumably due to *T. solium* larvae factors prevent inflammation [48].

The striking ability of helminth parasites in conferring protection from diseases of immune dysregulation has increased the attention into the immunomodulatory mechanisms evoked by these parasites. Administration of E-S antigens of *T. crassiceps* in experimental ulcerative colitis, autoimmune encephalomyelitis and type 1 diabetes shown positive results [49, 50]. The ability of *T. crassiceps* to prevent inflammatory responses was demonstrated to be dependent on a population of macrophages that produced markers of alternative activation (M2) [51]. Excreted/secreted *T. crassiceps* products decreased the production of inflammatory cytokines (IL-12, TNFα, and IL-6) in LPS-induced macrophages but has a limited role in inducing directly the production of M1 and/or M2-associated molecules. The immune-modulatory ability of these E-S antigens was further associated with increased levels of specific microRNAs, which are predicted to target numerous inflammatory mRNAs involved in the TNF and NF-κB signaling pathways [39].

3. miRNAs in drug response

In 2010 Devaney and collaborators [52] speculated that the link between changes in miRNA levels and drug resistance in cancer cells may also be a feature of drug resistance in parasitic nematodes. On the other hand, few data have been published in connection with drug resistance in cestodes [53]. Our group study the miRNA expression profile of *T. cr*assiceps cysticerci incubated for 24 h with sublethal doses of praziquantel (PZQ), one of the main antiparasitic agents used for cysticercosis and taeniasis [17].

The experiments showed that the overall miRNA profile remained unchanged under PZQ treatment, except for miR-7b that showed a sixfold enhanced expression [17] under PZQ treatment. One of the predicted miR- 7b targets was calponin, a calcium binding protein that inhibits myosin. This may be related to the expected alteration of intracellular calcium concentration produced by PZQ, a drug binding and inhibiting voltage-gated calcium channels, a key molecule for the regulation of calcium level inside the cell. Also, other targets of miR-7b are involved in several pathways such as amino acid and nucleotide metabolism, vesicular transport, signaling pathways, cell adhesion, cell growth, cell death and interaction with neuroactive ligands, suggesting the importance of this miRNA in parasite biology [17]. Calponin is one of miR- 7b predicted targets linked to calcium binding protein that inhibits myosin and may be related to the intracellular calcium concentration produced by PZQ. Other predicted targets of miR-7b are involved in several pathways such vesicular transport, signaling pathways, cell adhesion, cell growth, cell death and interaction with neuroactive ligands, suggesting the importance of this miRNA in parasite biology [17]. In these experiments other miRNAs showed differences in expression levels during treatment with PZQ, such as miR-31. This miRNA showed a decrease in the level of expression in cysticerci treated with PZQ and therefore the

Pathway	Gene ID	Description	miRNAs
Ion transporters	TsM_000896200	Voltage-gated calcium channel 2C	miR-307
	TsM_000896200	alpha-2 / delta	miR-36a
	TsM_000025300		miR-36b
	TsM_000025300		miR-124b
	TsM_000783500		miR-124a
	TsM_000896200		miR-133
	TsM_000436700		miR-745
	TsM_000598200		miR-31
	TsM_000845300		miR-2c
Drug metabolism / enzyme conjugation	TsM_000648500	Cytochrome b5-heme type /	miR-124a
	TsM_000648500	steroid binding	miR-124b
	TsM_000191900	Selenoprotein type 2C Rdx	miR-31
	TsM_000625200	Thioredoxin-like fold	miR-2a
	TsM_000625200	Glutathione S-transferase 2C	miR-2b
	TsM_000685100	class S	miR-9
	TsM_000979200	Thiolase-like	miR-281
	TsM_000610200	Glutathione S-transferase 2C	miR-307
	TsM_000860300	similar to C-terminal	miR-2162
	TsM_000219500		miR-96
ABC transporters	TsM_001160500	ABC type conveyors	miR-2b
	TsM_000989600	Type 2 ABC conveyors	miR-2c
	TsM_000971500	Type 1 2C ABC conveyors	miR-31
	TsM_001225200		miR-61
	TsM_000459700		miR-71
	TsM_000740200		miR-125
	TsM_000006800		miR-184
	TsM_000720400		miR-219
	TsM_000882500		miR-307
	TsM_000575300		miR-3479b
	TsM_000726600		

Table 2.
Interesting drug response miRNAs and targets in Taenia solium *genome.*

genes regulated by the miRNA would be overexpressed compared to the cysticerci that did not receive treatment with PZQ. Predicted target genes for this miRNA include: ABC transporters (transporters responsible for expelling different drugs out of the cell), thioredoxins (involved in drug metabolism), and the voltage-gated L-type calcium channel subunit alpha-1D, which is a probable site of action for praziquantel (PZQ) [54] **Table 2**. Additionally, other *T. solium* miRNAs were found to have targets related to flow, metabolism, and drug action [17].

These results prepare the way for continue with more studies in order to understand the response of miRNAs to drug treatment and the influence that these ncRNAs may have on drug action and/or drug resistance.

4. miRNAs as potential biomarkers

A biomarker is described as a feature that is objectively measured and evaluated as an indicator of many biological processes. Hunting for helminths biomarkers capable of providing diagnostic, prognostic, or therapeutic information has become a necessary but challenging work in cestodes research. MiRNAs were reported in blood – plasma, serum and other fluids like urine and saliva. This attribute has raised the interest of their use as potential biomarkers and diagnostic tools [55]. In the case of cestodes diseases the use of pathogen miRNAs as biomarkers promises the advent of highly specific and non-invasive diagnostic tools, since the miRNA repertoire of *T. solium* present a set of unique or divergent miRNAs with respect to the corresponding host homologs.

The small size and the stability of miRNAs are two important features that permit the circulation of these molecules in biological fluids. The formation of protein–miRNA allows circulating miRNAs escape of degradation [5]. Also, the majority of miRNAs detectable in serum and saliva are found inside extracellular vesicles (EV) that could avoid miRNA degradation and serve as transport particles to facilitate miRNA actions in neighboring cells [56]. The term EV groups includes several types of vesicles among which microvesicles and exosomes are the most thoroughly characterized. In helminths parasites EVs are the preferred extracellular compartment under study and miRNAs as the most thoroughly characterized RNA biotype [57]. The identification and sequencing of *T. solium* miRNAs is a must for their use as diagnostic tools. Among these contexts, the potential of miRNAs being involved in cestodes diseases as biomarkers has been investigated. It was demonstrated that the miR-10 and let-7 families are present in the EV from cestodes [57–61].
These two miRNAs are highly conserved throughout evolution and are present in bilaterians where they play fundamental roles in regulating stem-cell division and differentiation and embryonic development. The metacestode larval stage of *E. multilocularis* presents a morphological barrier to the secretion of EV towards the extra-parasite milieu and hence, ex-RNAs secreted in vitro are mostly detected in the EV-depleted fractions [57, 61]. Interestingly, the opposite is observed in the mestacestodes of *T crassiceps* and *M. vagae*, a parasites models of *T. solium*, that do not have such a structure [61] but parasite ex-RNA detection in patient biofluids is still in a very early phase of study.

The extensive use of next generation of technologies such as miRNA microarrays and high-throughput deep sequencing techniques, translating biomarker into practice with increased diagnostic and therapeutic sensitivity and specificity would be less of a problem [62]. With respect to the use of ex-RNAs as biomarkers in NCC, to date, no laboratory assay from plasma, serum or cerebrospinal fluid has been performed. Furthermore, patient samples from different geographic regions together with specificity assessment with samples of patients would also provide a more realistic view of the potential of ex-RNAs as biomarkers of NCC.

5. miRNAs as potential drug target

The hypothesis that many *T. solium* miRNAs have crucial roles in development, host–parasite interaction and immune response, and also the absent of some miRNAs in the host has led to considerable interest in the therapeutic targeting of miRNAs in NCC. The main approaches commonly taken are: i) miRNA inhibition by antisense oligonucleotides, miRNA sponges or small-molecule inhibitors ii) miRNA upregulation with miRNA mimics [63]. Mirna sponges' strategies rely on the expression of mRNAs containing multiple artificial miRNA-binding sites, which act as decoys. The overexpression of mRNA- sponges selectively sequesters endogenous miRNAs and thus allows expression of the target mRNAs [64]. Approaches that are based on small molecules generally rely on reporter-based assay systems for compound library screening and have identified small molecules that could specifically inhibit miRNA expression, such as azobenzene (which affects human miR-21 expression) and several diverse compounds that inhibit human miR-122 [65]. Considerably more attention has been paid to antimiRs, particularly to those that target miRNAs directly to specifically inhibit miRNA function and upregulate miRNA targets. In practice chemical modification of oligonucleotides is required to increase resistance to serum nucleases, to enhance binding affinity for targeted miRNAs and to improve the pharmacokinetics and pharmacodynamics profile in vivo. Other limitations are associated with rapid clearance, immunotoxicity an low tissue permeability. The delivery of artificial miRNAs or of blocking counterparts that could interfere with key processes in parasites has been already postulated by several authors, and some potential targets are already characterized. MiRNA manipulation in parasites has been also proposed as a new strategy for control against schistosomiasis and cystic echinococcosis [38, 66].

6. Conclusions

For the better understand of the pathophysiology of parasitic diseases at the molecular level is crucial identify and characterize parasite-specific miRNAs and their targets in hosts. The significant advance in biomedical research of miRNAs as target drugs and biomarkers is expected to be widely translated in the field of parasitology in the coming years. Why not think about miRNAs as a profitable approach to better diagnose and properly treat NNC? There is an increasing number of studies that are being done in *T. solium* and cestodes miRNAs, however translational research of miRNA still remains a challenge.

Regarding the neglected diseases, researchers have dedicated decades to the development of new drugs and identifying new biomarkers of disease progression but most researches are limited to academia indicating a gap between basic science and clinical application. Also, the use of miRNAs as a biomarker or potential drug target are poorly explored compared with cancer, neurological disorders, metabolic, cardiac and circulatory diseases.

It is expected that in future years the biological knowledge acquired on miRNAs, especially in biomedical research, could be widely translated into NNC since miRNAs could hold great potential as therapeutic and diagnosis targets for the control of diseases.

Acknowledgments

I would like to thanks Dr. Mara Rosenzvit and all the members of the BMHid laboratory (https://impam.conicet.gov.ar/bmhid/).

Author details

Matías Gastón Pérez
Institute for Research in Medical Microbiology and Parasitology (IMPaM-UBA-CONICET), Buenos Aires, Argentina

*Address all correspondence to: mgperez@fvet.uba.ar; matiasperez@conicet.gov.ar

References

[1] Bartel DP. MicroRNAs: genomics, biogenesis, mechanism, and function. Cell. 2004;116(2):281-297. doi:10.1016/s0092-8674(04)00045-5.

[2] Lee RC, Feinbaum RL, Ambros V. The *C. elegans* heterochronic gene lin-4 encodes small RNAs with antisense complementarity to lin-14. Cell. 1993;75(5):843-854. doi:10.1016/0092-8674(93)90529-y.

[3] Pasquinelli AE, Reinhart BJ, Slack F, et al. Conservation of the sequence and temporal expression of let-7 heterochronic regulatory RNA. Nature. 2000;408(6808):86-89. doi:10.1038/35040556.

[4] Bartel DP. Metazoan MicroRNAs. Cell. 2018;173(1):20-51. doi: 10.1016/j.cell.2018.03.006.

[5] O'Brien J, Hayder H, Zayed Y, Peng C. Overview of MicroRNA Biogenesis, Mechanisms of Actions, and Circulation. Front Endocrinol (Lausanne). 2018; 9:402. Published 2018 Aug 3. doi:10.3389/fendo.2018.00402.

[6] Liu B, Shyr Y, Cai J, Liu Q. Interplay between miRNAs and host genes and their role in cancer. Brief Funct Genomics. 2018;18(4):255-266. doi:10.1093/bfgp/elz002.

[7] Ha M, Kim VN. Regulation of microRNA biogenesis. Nat Rev Mol Cell Biol. 2014;15(8):509-524. doi:10.1038/nrm3838.

[8] Guo L, Chen F. A challenge for miRNA: multiple isomiRs in miRNAomics. Gene. 2014;544(1):1-7. doi: 10.1016/j.gene.2014.04.039.

[9] Kozomara A, Griffiths-Jones S. miRBase: integrating microRNA annotation and deep-sequencing data. Nucleic Acids Res. 2011;39(Database issue):D152-D157. doi:10.1093/nar/gkq1027.

[10] Bartel DP. MicroRNAs: target recognition and regulatory functions. Cell. 2009;136(2):215-233. doi:10.1016/j.cell.2009.01.002.

[11] Mathelier A, Carbone A. Large scale chromosomal mapping of human microRNA structural clusters. Nucleic Acids Res. 2013;41(8):4392-4408. doi:10.1093/nar/gkt112.

[12] Kamanu TK, Radovanovic A, Archer JA, Bajic VB. Exploration of miRNA families for hypotheses generation. Sci Rep. 2013; 3:2940. Published 2013 Oct 15. doi:10.1038/srep02940.

[13] Ha M, Kim VN. Regulation of microRNA biogenesis. Nat Rev Mol Cell Biol. 2014;15(8):509-524. doi:10.1038/nrm3838.

[14] Petrovic N, Ergun S. miRNAs as Potential Treatment Targets and Treatment Options in Cancer. Mol Diagn Ther. 2018;22(2):157-168. doi:10.1007/s40291-017-0314-8.

[15] Chakraborty C, Sharma AR, Sharma G, Lee SS. Therapeutic advances of miRNAs: A preclinical and clinical update. J Adv Res. 2020; 28:127-138. Published 2020 Aug 29. doi: 10.1016/j.jare.2020.08.012.

[16] Tsai IJ, Zarowiecki M, Holroyd N, et al. The genomes of four tapeworm species reveal adaptations to parasitism. Nature. 2013;496(7443):57-63. doi:10.1038/nature12031.

[17] Pérez MG, Macchiaroli N, Lichtenstein G, et al. microRNA analysis of *Taenia crassiceps* cysticerci under praziquantel treatment and genome-wide identification of *Taenia solium* miRNAs. Int J Parasitol.

2017;47(10-11):643-653. doi: 10.1016/j. ijpara.2017.04.002.

[18] Cucher M, Prada L, Mourglia-Ettlin G, et al. Identification of *Echinococcus granulosus* microRNAs and their expression in different life cycle stages and parasite genotypes. Int J Parasitol. 2011;41(3-4):439-448. doi: 10.1016/j.ijpara.2010.11.010.

[19] Winter AD, Weir W, Hunt M, et al. Diversity in parasitic nematode genomes: the microRNAs of *Brugia pahangi* and *Haemonchus contortus* are largely novel. BMC Genomics. 2012; 13:4. Published 2012 Jan 4. doi:10.1186/1471-2164-13-4.

[20] Macchiaroli N, Cucher M, Zarowiecki M, Maldonado L, Kamenetzky L, Rosenzvit MC. microRNA profiling in the zoonotic parasite *Echinococcus canadensis* using a high-throughput approach. Parasit Vectors. 2015;8:83. Published 2015 Feb 6. doi:10.1186/s13071-015-0686-8.

[21] Basika T, Macchiaroli N, Cucher M, et al. Identification and profiling of microRNAs in two developmental stages of the model cestode parasite *Mesocestoides corti*. Mol Biochem Parasitol. 2016;210(1-2):37-49. doi:10.1016/j.molbiopara.2016.08.004.

[22] Fromm B, Worren MM, Hahn C, Hovig E, Bachmann L. Substantial loss of conserved and gain of novel MicroRNA families in flatworms. Mol Biol Evol. 2013;30(12):2619-2628. doi:10.1093/molbev/mst155.

[23] Bai Y, Zhang Z, Jin L, et al. Genome-wide sequencing of small RNAs reveals a tissue-specific loss of conserved microRNA families in *Echinococcus granulosus*. BMC Genomics. 2014;15(1):736. Published 2014 Aug 29. doi:10.1186/1471-2164-15-736.

[24] Cucher M, Macchiaroli N, Kamenetzky L, Maldonado L, Brehm K, Rosenzvit MC. High-throughput characterization of *Echinococcus* spp. metacestode miRNomes. Int J Parasitol. 2015;45(4):253-267. doi: 10.1016/j. ijpara.2014.12.003.

[25] Lee YS, Dutta A. MicroRNAs in cancer. Annu Rev Pathol. 2009; 4:199-227. doi: 10.1146/annurev. pathol.4.110807.092222.

[26] Kabekkodu SP, Shukla V, Varghese VK, D' Souza J, Chakrabarty S, Satyamoorthy K. Clustered miRNAs and their role in biological functions and diseases. Biol Rev Camb Philos Soc. 2018;93(4):1955-1986. doi:10.1111/ brv.12428.

[27] Landa A, Navarro L, Ochoa-Sánchez A, Jiménez L. *Taenia solium* and *Taenia crassiceps*: miRNomes of the larvae and effects of miR-10-5p and let-7-5p on murine peritoneal macrophages. Biosci Rep. 2019;39(11): BSR20190152. doi:10.1042/ BSR20190152.

[28] Cai P, Hou N, Piao X, et al. Profiles of small non-coding RNAs in *Schistosoma japonicum* during development. PLoS Negl Trop Dis. 2011;5(8): e1256. doi: 10.1371/journal. pntd.0001256.

[29] Zhi F, Shao N, Wang R, et al. Identification of 9 serum microRNAs as potential noninvasive biomarkers of human astrocytoma. Neuro Oncol. 2015;17(3):383-391. doi:10.1093/ neuonc/nou169.

[30] Giusti J, Pinhal D, Moxon S, Campos CL, Münsterberg A, Martins C. MicroRNA-10 modulates Hox genes expression during Nile tilapia embryonic development. Mech Dev. 2016;140:12-18. doi: 10.1016/j. mod.2016.03.002.

[31] Mansfield JH, McGlinn E. Evolution, expression, and developmental function of

Hox-embedded miRNAs. Curr Top Dev Biol. 2012; 99:31-57. doi:10.1016/B978-0-12-387038-4.00002-1.

[32] Reinhart BJ, Slack FJ, Basson M, et al. The 21-nucleotide let-7 RNA regulates developmental timing in *Caenorhabditis elegans*. Nature. 2000;403(6772):901-906. doi:10.1038/35002607.

[33] Zhu H, Shyh-Chang N, Segrè AV, et al. The Lin28/let-7 axis regulates glucose metabolism. Cell. 2011;147(1):81-94. doi: 10.1016/j.cell.2011.08.033

[34] Pérez MG, Spiliotis M, Rego N, et al. Deciphering the role of miR-71 in *Echinococcus multilocularis* early development in vitro. PLoS Negl Trop Dis. 2019;13(12):e0007932. Published 2019 Dec 27. doi: 10.1371/journal.pntd.0007932.

[35] Maizels RM, Smits HH, McSorley HJ. Modulation of Host Immunity by Helminths: The Expanding Repertoire of Parasite Effector Molecules. Immunity. 2018;49(5):801-818. doi:10.1016/j.immuni.2018.10.016.

[36] Sikasunge CS, Johansen MV, Phiri IK, Willingham AL 3rd, Leifsson PS. The immune response in *Taenia solium* neurocysticercosis in pigs is associated with astrogliosis, axonal degeneration and altered blood-brain barrier permeability. Vet Parasitol. 2009;160(3-4):242-250. doi:10.1016/j.vetpar.2008.11.015

[37] Fleury, A., Cardenas, G., Adalid-Peralta, L., Fragoso, G., and Sciutto, E. Immunopathology in *Taenia solium* neurocysticercosis. Parasite Immunol. 2016; 38, 147-157. doi: 10.1111/pim.12299.

[38] Rouas, R., Fayyad-Kazan, H., El Zein, N., Lewalle, P., Rothé, F., Simion, A., Akl, H., Mourtada, M., El Rifai, M., Burny, A., Romero, P., Martiat, P., Badran, B. Human natural Treg microRNA signature: role of microRNA-31 and microRNA21 in FOXP3 expression. Eur. J. Immunol. 2009; 39, 1608-1618.

[39] Martínez-Saucedo D, Ruíz-Rosado JD, Terrazas C, Callejas BE, Satoskar AR, Partida-Sánchez S, Terrazas LI. *Taenia crassiceps*-Excreted/Secreted Products Induce a Defined MicroRNA Profile that Modulates Inflammatory Properties of Macrophages. J Immunol Res. 2019 May 14;2019:2946713. doi: 10.1155/2019/2946713.

[40] Curtale G, Rubino M, Locati M. MicroRNAs as Molecular Switches in Macrophage Activation. Front Immunol. 2019;10:799. Published 2019 Apr 17. doi:10.3389/fimmu.2019.00799.

[41] Davidson-Moncada, J., Papavasiliou, F. N., and Tam, W. MicroRNAs of the immune system. Ann. N.Y. Acad. Sci. 2010; 1183, 183-194. doi: 10.1111/j.1749-6632.2009.05121.

[42] Atri C, Guerfali FZ, Laouini D. Role of Human Macrophage Polarization in Inflammation during Infectious Diseases. Int J Mol Sci. 2018;19(6):1801. Published 2018 Jun 19. doi:10.3390/ijms19061801.

[43] Peón AN, Espinoza-Jiménez A, Terrazas LI. Immunoregulation by *Taenia crassiceps* and its antigens. Biomed Res Int. 2013;2013:498583. doi:10.1155/2013/498583.

[44] Reyes JL, Terrazas CA, Vera-Arias L, Terrazas LI. Differential response of antigen presenting cells from susceptible and resistant strains of mice to *Taenia crassiceps* infection. Infect Genet Evol. 2009;9(6):1115-1127. doi:10.1016/j.meegid.2009.05.011.

[45] Rothaug M, Becker-Pauly C, Rose-John S. The role of interleukin-6 signaling in nervous tissue. Biochim

Biophys Acta. 2016;1863(6 Pt A):1218-1227. doi:10.1016/j.bbamcr.2016.03.018.

[46] Probert L. TNF and its receptors in the CNS: The essential, the desirable and the deleterious effects. Neuroscience. 2015;302:2-22. doi:10.1016/j.neuroscience.2015.06.038.

[47] Mahanty S, Orrego MA, Mayta H, et al. Post-treatment vascular leakage and inflammatory responses around brain cysts in porcine neurocysticercosis. PLoS Negl Trop Dis. 2015;9(3): e0003577. Published 2015 Mar 16. doi:10.1371/journal.pntd.0003577.

[48] Fleury A, Cardenas G, Adalid-Peralta L, Fragoso G, Sciutto E. Immunopathology in *Taenia solium* neurocysticercosis. Parasite Immunol. 2016;38(3):147-157. doi:10.1111/pim.12299.

[49] Peón AN, Ledesma-Soto Y, Olguín JE, Bautista-Donis M, Sciutto E, Terrazas LI. Helminth Products Potently Modulate Experimental Autoimmune Encephalomyelitis by Downregulating Neuroinflammation and Promoting a Suppressive Microenvironment. Mediators Inflamm. 2017;2017: 8494572. doi:10.1155/2017/8494572.

[50] Ledesma-Soto Y, Callejas BE, Terrazas CA, et al. Extraintestinal Helminth Infection Limits Pathology and Proinflammatory Cytokine Expression during DSS-Induced Ulcerative Colitis: A Role for Alternatively Activated Macrophages and Prostaglandins. Biomed Res Int. 2015;2015:563425. doi:10.1155/2015/563425.

[51] Rehli M., Sulzbacher S., Pape S., et al. Transcription factor Tfec contributes to the IL-4-inducible expression of a small group of genes in mouse macrophages including the granulocyte colony-stimulating factor receptor. The Journal of Immunology. 2005;174(11):7111-7122. doi: 10.4049/jimmunol.174.11.7111.

[52] Devaney E, Winter AD, Britton C. microRNAs: a role in drug resistance in parasitic nematodes? Trends Parasitol. 2010;26(9):428-433. doi:10.1016/j.pt.2010.05.003.

[53] Jesudoss Chelladurai J, Kifleyohannes T, Scott J, Brewer MT. Praziquantel Resistance in the Zoonotic Cestode *Dipylidium caninum*. Am J Trop Med Hyg. 2018;99(5):1201-1205. doi:10.4269/ajtmh.18-0533.

[54] Greenberg RM. Ca2+ signalling, voltage-gated Ca2+ channels and praziquantel in flatworm neuromusculature. Parasitology. 2005;131 Suppl:S97-108. doi: 10.1017/S0031182005008346.

[55] Condrat CE, Thompson DC, Barbu MG, et al. miRNAs as Biomarkers in Disease: Latest Findings Regarding Their Role in Diagnosis and Prognosis. Cells. 2020;9(2):276. doi:10.3390/cells9020276.

[56] Boon RA, Iekushi K, Lechner S, Seeger T, Fischer A, Heydt S, Kaluza D, Tréguer K, Carmona G, Bonauer A, Horrevoets AJ, Didier N, Girmatsion Z, Biliczki P, Ehrlich JR, Katus HA, Müller OJ, Potente M, Zeiher AM, Hermeking H, Dimmeler S. MicroRNA-34a regulates cardiac ageing and function. Nature. 2013 Mar 7;495(7439):107-10. doi: 10.1038/nature11919. Epub 2013 Feb 20. PMID: 23426265.

[57] Ancarola ME, Lichtenstein G, Herbig J, et al. Extracellular non-coding RNA signatures of the metacestode stage of *Echinococcus multilocularis*. PLoS Negl Trop Dis. 2020;14(11): e0008890. Published 2020 Nov 30. doi:10.1371/journal.pntd.0008890.

[58] Ding J, He G, Wu J, et al. miRNA-seq of *Echinococcus multilocularis* Extracellular Vesicles and Immunomodulatory Effects of miR-4989. Front Microbiol. 2019;10:2707. Published 2019 Nov 29. doi:10.3389/fmicb.2019.02707.

[59] Liang P, Mao L, Zhang S, et al. Identification and molecular characterization of exosome-like vesicles derived from the *Taenia asiatica* adult worm. Acta Trop. 2019;198:105036. doi:10.1016/j.actatropica.2019.05.027

[60] Wang L, Li Z, Shen J, et al. Exosome-like vesicles derived by *Schistosoma japonicum* adult worms mediates M1 type immune- activity of macrophage. Parasitol Res. 2015;114(5):1865-1873. doi:10.1007/s00436-015-4373-7.

[61] Ancarola ME, Marcilla A, Herz M, et al. Cestode parasites release extracellular vesicles with microRNAs and immunodiagnostic protein cargo. Int J Parasitol. 2017;47(10-11):675-686. doi:10.1016/j.ijpara.2017.05.003.

[62] Tribolet L, Kerr E, Cowled C, et al. MicroRNA Biomarkers for Infectious Diseases: From Basic Research to Biosensing. Front Microbiol. 2020;11:1197. Published 2020 Jun 3. doi:10.3389/fmicb.2020.01197.

[63] Broderick JA, Zamore PD. MicroRNA therapeutics. Gene Ther. 2011;18(12):1104-1110. doi:10.1038/gt.2011.50.

[64] Baumann V, Winkler J. miRNA-based therapies: strategies and delivery platforms for oligonucleotide and non-oligonucleotide agents. Future Med Chem. 2014;6(17):1967-1984. doi:10.4155/fmc.14.116

[65] Ryoo JH, Wang C, Swearer SM, Hull M, Shi D. Longitudinal Model Building Using Latent Transition Analysis: An Example Using School Bullying Data. Front Psychol. 2018;9:675. Published 2018 May 8. doi:10.3389/fpsyg.2018.00675.

[66] Paul S, Ruiz-Manriquez LM, Serrano-Cano FI, Estrada-Meza C, Solorio-Diaz KA, Srivastava A. Human microRNAs in host-parasite interaction: a review. 3 Biotech. 2020;10(12):510. doi:10.1007/s13205-020-02498-6.

Chapter 6

Development of New Drugs to Treat *Taenia solium* Cysticercosis: Targeting 26 kDa Glutathione Transferase

Rafael A. Zubillaga, Lucía Jiménez,
Ponciano García-Gutiérrez and Abraham Landa

Abstract

Taenia solium causes neurocysticercosis, a parasitic infection of the central nervous system in humans. The costs of management, treatment, and diagnosis of patients with neurocysticercosis are high, and some patients do not respond to the currently available treatments. Helminth cytosolic glutathione transferases (GSTs) are essential enzymes involved in the regulation of immune responses, transport, and detoxification. In *T. solium*, three cytosolic GSTs with molecular masses of 26.5 (Ts26GST), 25.5 (Ts25GST), and 24.3 kDa (TsMσGST), classified as mu-alpha, mu and sigma GST-classes, respectively, constitute the main detoxification system, and they may be immune targets for the development of vaccines and new anthelmintics. We performed a successful virtual screen, and identified I7, a novel selective inhibitor of Ts26GST that showed a non-competitive inhibition mechanism towards substrate glutathione with a Ki of 55.7 mM and mixed inhibition towards the electrophilic substrate 1-chloro-2,4-dinitrobenzene with a Ki of 8.64 mM. Docking simulation studies showed that I7 can bind to a site that is adjacent to the electrophilic site and the furthest from the glutathione site. This new inhibitor of Ts26GST will be used as a lead molecule to develop new effective and safe drugs against diseases caused by *T. solium*.

Keywords: Glutathione transferase, Inhibitor, *Taenia solium*, Neurocysticercosis

1. Introduction

1.1 Neurocysticercosis

Taenia solium is a cestode parasite in humans. Adult parasites cause taeniasis, and the larvae cause cysticercosis. Larvae located in the central nervous system cause neurocysticercosis (NCC), with a wide spectrum of clinical manifestations that depend on factors such as the location, number of larvae, and the intensity of host immune response [1, 2]. The disease may be asymptomatic or present with nonspecific symptoms, such as epilepsy, cognitive impairment, migraine-type headache, intracranial hypertension, and neurological deficits, among other symptoms [3, 4].

1.2 Clinical spectrum

According to the location of the larvae, NCC is classified into parenchymal NCC and extraparenchymal NCC. In the parenchymal NCC, the most frequent symptoms are seizures, which can occur at any stage of the cysticercus (viable or calcified) [5], and neurological signs, such as sensory deficits, language, and gait disturbances, as well as involuntary movements. Such manifestations have been reported in up to 15% of patients [3]. In the extraparenchymal NCC, cysticerci are usually found in the subarachnoid and ventricular locations. Hydrocephalus is observed in a significant number of cases of subarachnoid NCC, and neurological alterations associated with the obstruction of the cerebrospinal fluid flow have been observed in patients with ventricular NCC; the blockage of the cerebral aqueduct due to the presence of cysticerci in the fourth ventricle may result in the loss of consciousness or even death [3, 6, 7].

1.3 Treatment

NCC is a disease transmitted by food, which causes many disability-adjusted life years. In Mexico, the cost of management, treatment, and diagnosis of patients with NCC was approximately U.S. $52 million in 2015 [8]. In addition to these costs, a study in Peru estimated that two-thirds of patients who develop symptoms lose their jobs, and the sequelae make it impossible for 60% of them to return to work [9]. Treatment should be individualized according to the characteristics of the disease and location of cysticerci, but in general, it consists of a mixture of surgical intervention (recommended for cases of intraventricular or spinal NCC), antiparasitic and anti-inflammatory drugs, and drugs for the management of symptoms [10]. The antiparasitic treatment for NCC includes praziquantel or albendazole. Praziquantel is a pyrazino-isoquinoline derivative that affects calcium channels on the parasite's surface and causes muscle contractions, paralysis, and tegument damage [11]. Maximum serum levels of praziquantel are obtained in 1.5–2 h after administration [12]. Praziquantel is metabolized in the liver, and its mild side effects include gastric disturbances, dizziness, drowsiness, fever, headache, increased sweating, and sometimes allergic reactions; however, these reactions disappear when the drug is withdrawn [13]. Albendazole is a benzimidazole compound that leads to the selective degeneration of cytoplasmic microtubules, affecting the formation of ATP, and glucose intake, which depletes parasite of the energy source [14]. Maximum serum levels of albendazole are achieved in 2 to 3 h after ingestion. This drug penetrates the cerebrospinal fluid better than praziquantel [15]. Side effects in humans are mainly related to liver toxicity (increased liver enzymes), hematological effects, hair loss, and general symptoms that dissipate when treatment is withdrawn [14]. The use of antiparasitic drugs can cause adverse effects arising from the inflammatory reaction induced when cysticerci are damaged; therefore, the use of corticosteroids in addition to treatment is recommended. However, prolonged use of corticosteroids increases the risk of opportunistic infections, skin disorders, depression, osteopenia, among others [13]. Several drugs, including benzimidazole, praziquantel and nitazoxanide, have been evaluated for their ability to control swine cysticercosis in animals intended for consumption. Of these, oxfendazole has been shown to have close to 100% efficacy after a single dose in intramuscular cysticercosis, but the efficacy was lower in swine neurocysticercosis [16].

1.4 New drugs

Patients who do not respond to therapy with the currently available drugs have been reported. Several factors have been proposed that may be involved in this lack of sensitivity to the treatment: differential response according to the state of development of cysticerci, low penetration of the drug into the subarachnoid space, variability of albendazole sulfoxide levels in plasma in individual patients, or interference of corticosteroids with the activity of anti-helmintics [17, 18]. This has led to the search for new drugs that could improve the effectiveness of the anti-helminthic therapy. Therefore, cytosolic glutathione transferases (cGSTs) have been selected as targets for the development of vaccines and drugs against this parasite [19–22].

2. Overview of glutathione transferases

2.1 The catalytic reaction

GSTs (EC 2.5.1.18) are a multiprotein family highly expressed in all cells [23, 24]. They are part of phase II detoxification process and catalyze the conjugation of glutathione to a variety of endo- and exo-electrophilic substrates [25]. This conjugation produces soluble compounds and substrates for cellular export proteins, such as P-glycoprotein and multidrug resistance-related protein 1 [26]. The general reactions (GSH + RX → GSR + HX) comprise a nucleophilic attack, aromatic substitution, epoxide ring opening, reversible Michael addition, isomerization or peroxidation. Although nucleophilic attack can also be directed to nitrogen atoms in nitrate esters, sulfurs in organic thiocyanates or disulfites, and oxygen in organic hydroperoxides [25, 27–29].

2.2 Cellular distribution and GST classes

GSTs can be grouped into three subfamilies according to their cellular location: mitochondrial GSTs, microsomal GSTs or MAPEGs (membrane-associated proteins in eicosanoid and GSH metabolism), and cytosolic or canonical GSTs. In humans, genes encoding all expressed GSTs from a given subfamily are clustered on the same chromosome [30]. The mitochondrial GST subfamily includes a unique kappa (K) class. This class has very high peroxidase activity, and its location suggests an important role in β-oxidation of fatty acids and in lipid peroxidation. Moreover, it is also a key regulator of adiponectin biosynthesis and may function as a chaperone [31–34]. Microsomal GSTs are divided into four groups (I–IV). They share less than 20% sequence identity and are involved in eicosanoid metabolism, such as the synthesis of prostaglandins, thromboxanes, leukotrienes (inhibitors of inflammation), glutathione metabolism, and activation of some lipoxygenases [33, 35–37]. In the subfamily of cGSTs, members of the same class have more than 40% amino acid sequence identity, whereas sequence identity between classes is below 25%. cGSTs are divided into: (1) organism-specific GST classes, which include several GSTs, such as lambda (L), phi (F), and tau (U) in plants; delta (D), epsilon (E) in insects; beta (B) in prokaryotes; and 2) ubiquitous classes in any organism, including mu (M), alpha (A), pi (P), theta (T), sigma (S), zeta (Z), and omega (O) classes. Each of them displays distinct catalytic and non-catalytic binding properties, and their functions are very versatile and involve detoxification, signal modulation, catabolism of aromatic amino acids, ion channel modulation, chemotherapy resistance, prostaglandin and steroid hormone synthesis, and transport of molecules such as bilirubin, heme, steroids, hormones, and bile salts [25, 27, 29, 31, 33, 38–43].

2.3 Structural characteristics

All cGSTs are dimers with 24–27 kDa monomeric subunits containing ~250 amino acid residues on average. They share the same tertiary and quaternary structures, and each subunit has two distinct functional domains. The first domain is the G site, which is located at the N-terminal region and is responsible for GSH binding. This domain is highly conserved in all classes and has a thioredoxin-like fold constructed by three helices and four sheets (βαβαββα). Activation of GSH occurs at the G-site by different amino acids, depending on the class, and is either a tyrosine (Y) found in M, P, A, and S-classes, a serine (S) found in T, Z, F, U, and D-classes, or a cysteine (C) to O, and B-classes. The activation allows a nucleophilic attack on the electrophilic compounds, allowing conjugation or thiol transfer. The first two amino acids, tyrosine and serine, promote the formation and stabilization of the thiolate anion of GSH, lowering its pKa to 6.2. This is achieved through hydrogen bond donation of the hydroxyl group, which makes GSH ready for conjugation. The C residue is used for thiol transfer, and it forms mixed disulfides with GSH. The N-terminal domain consensus sequence SNAIL/TRAIL is localized in the region between residues 68 and 77, and appears in all mammalian cGSTs [25, 29, 31, 44, 45]. The second domain is the H site, which is localized in the C-terminal region. This domain binds the electrophilic substrate, and it is constituted exclusively by α-helices. The number of helices varies from four to seven, depending on the class. This variation has been used to explain the wide range of electrophilic substrates for detoxification and specificity among classes. For example, the M-class has very efficient catalysis with molecules containing oxiranes and unsaturated carbonyl groups, whereas A-class acts on 4-hydroxyalkenals and peroxides [20, 25, 31, 33, 45]. Although GSTs do not present specificity for their hydrophobic substrates, they seem very specific for the γ-glutamyl portion of GSH, and there is evidence that a peptide portion in the conjugate binds to ATP pumps or the multidrug resistance-associated proteins to be exported [46, 47]. Furthermore, in these domains, there are also conserved motifs that identify GST classes. For example, the primary and secondary structures that form the mu-loop or α9-helix are characteristic of M, and A-GST classes [20, 45, 48].

2.4 Alternative functions of GSTs

Besides their catalytic role, ligandin activity has been identified in GSTs because they bind toxic non-substrate ligands, such as hemin, bilirubin, bile salts, steroids, thyroid hormones, fatty acids, drugs (albendazole and praziquantel), and members of the MAPK protein kinase family, which are involved in processes such as the production, storage, and rapid transport of prostaglandins out of cells, intrinsic and acquired drug resistance, cell survival and apoptosis, contributing to passive detoxification or intracellular transport in cells. The ligandin site is different from the G and H sites, and the above-mentioned toxic non-substrates are able to inhibit the catalytic activity of GSTs [49–52]. Another striking property of the GST enzyme is its translocation from the outside to the inside of various cells. This internalization occurs through endocytosis mediated by receptors or by the GST-fold structure, and it is independent of GST function as an enzyme [53, 54].

2.5 GSTs in platyhelminthes

In these parasites, GSTs also act as xenobiotic detoxifying enzymes, catalyzing conjugation of GSH (active detoxification) or, in the case of ligandin, transporting toxic substrates (passive detoxification) and acting as protective antigens to the host [23, 55]. Finally, many reports on vaccination experiments have described reductions in parasite burden, fecal egg counts, tissue egg densities, and female fecundity in experimental cysticercosis, schistosomiasis, and fascioliasis [23, 56–60]. The World Health Organization has recommended the use of *Schistosoma japonicum*

GST (SjGST) as a vaccine antigen in the form of a DNA vaccine (pcDNA/sjGST) in nanoparticles combined with pIL-12 [61, 62].

2.6 GSTs in *T. solium*

In the cestode *T. solium*, GST activity has been identified in the microsomal fraction, and it was noncompetitively inhibited by triphenyltin chloride and bromosulfophthalein [63]. Moreover, three cGSTs classes have been identified according to the classification of mammalian GSTs [20]: (i) a moderately abundant S-class GST denoted as TsMσGST, (ii) the least abundant M-class GST named Ts25GST (previously referred to as SGSTM1), which has a high capacity to conjugate reactive carbonyls, the secondary products of lipid peroxidation, and (iii) the most abundant M and A-class GST named Ts26GST (previously referred to as SGSTM2). The characteristics and properties of these enzymes are listed in **Table 1**.

The specific antibodies produced against each TsGST (TsMσGST, Ts25GST, and Ts26GST) showed that they are not antigenically related to each other, nor to trematode, cestode, or mammalian GSTs [19, 20, 64]. Interestingly, these specific antibodies recognized the homologous GST class in *T. saginata*, *T. taeniaeformis*, and *T. crassiceps*. On the other hand, immunizations of a murine model of cysticercosis with the SGSTF fraction purified from cysticerci (comprising both Ts25GST and Ts26GST) or with recombinant Ts26GST alone were highly effective in reducing cysticerci load by 90% and 74%, respectively, whereas the use of the native and recombinant Ts25GST as immunogens afforded lower protection rates, 46% and 25%, respectively [19].

The aforementioned result as well as the known lack of catalase and low activities of CYP450 and glutathione peroxidase have led us to postulate that GSTs are the major detoxification system for this parasite. In addition, the properties of cGSTs as immunogens and vaccination candidates make them attractive targets for the development of new drugs against this parasite [19, 20, 22, 64].

Anti-helminthic compounds such as mebendazole and praziquantel inhibited Ts26GST and TsMσGST *in vitro*, but they did not reach plasma concentrations *in vivo* that would allow effective inhibition of enzyme activity [20, 64, 65, 66]. To date, a

	TsMσGST	Ts25GST	Ts26GST
Number of amino acids	212	219	221
Molecular mass (Da)	24,290	25,496	25,936
Number of isoforms	4	2	4
Isoelectric point	8.2–8.7	5.7–6.3	7.2–8.5
V_{max}(CDNB) (μmol min^{-1} mg^{-1})	1.08	12.0	51.5
K_M(CDNB) (mM)	0.16	1.38	1.06
V_{max}(GSH) (μmol min^{-1} mg^{-1})	0.78	10.2	39.9
K_M(GSH) (mM)	0.17	0.905	0.20
Classes of effective inhibitors	A, M	A, M	A, M
Optimal conditions	pH 8.0, 40 °C	pH 8.0, 37–40°C	pH 7-5, 37–40°C
Main location	Scolex	Tegument, and parenchyma	Tegument, and parenchyma

Table 1.
Cytosolic glutathione transferases from Taenia solium.

non-toxic inhibitor for GST has not been developed, but ethacrynic acid, haloenol lactone, disulfiram, and curcumin are potent inhibitors of human GST-P1 [67, 68]. A new generation of drugs, such as modified ethacrynic acid, γ-glutamyl-S-(benzyl) cysteinyl-R(−)-phenyl glycine diethyl ester (TER 199), and prodrug (TER 286), provide a starting point for development of novel powerful and specific inhibitors against human GST-P1. However, the clinical side effects have limited their application [24].

3. Kinetic and structural properties of Ts26GST

3.1 Kinetic mechanism of Ts26GST in the CDNB conjugation reaction

Ts26GST is a bisustrate enzyme that exhibits a higher affinity for glutathione (GSH) than for 1-chloro-2,4-dinitrobenzene (CDNB), unlike other two cGSTs of

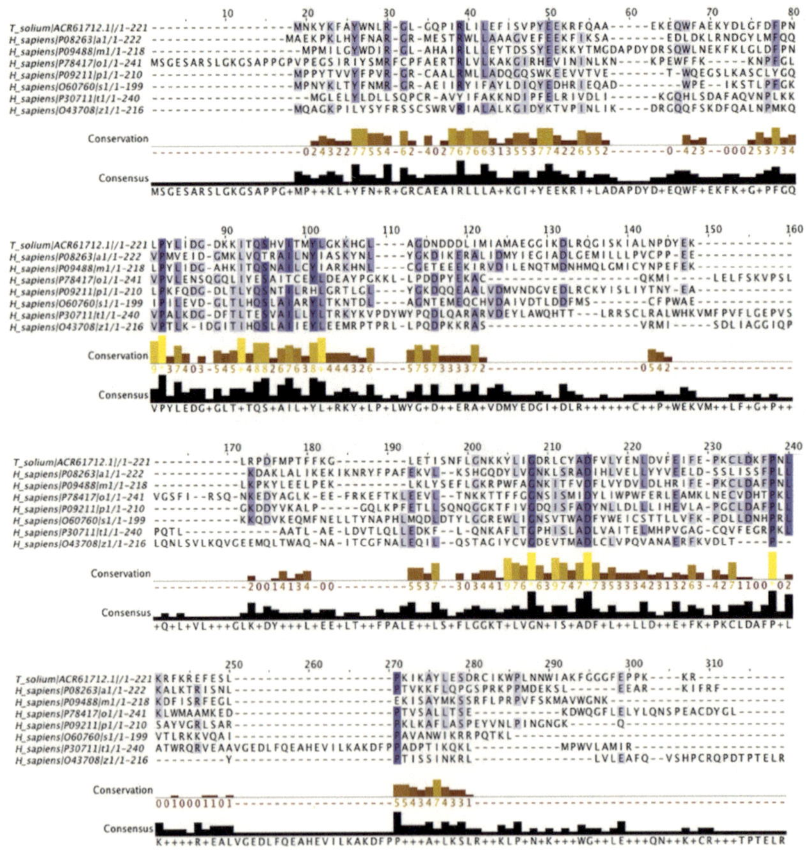

Percent Identity Matrix (created by Clustal 2.1

1: T_solium|ACR61712.1|	100.00	26.79	41.78	17.22	26.47	24.34	16.84	16.36
2: H_sapiens|P08263|a1	26.79	100.00	23.76	22.40	28.99	25.26	16.32	21.76
3: H_sapiens|P09488|m1	41.78	23.76	100.00	19.08	28.71	25.93	19.25	14.56
4: H_sapiens|P78417|o1	17.22	22.40	19.08	100.00	20.59	21.05	18.65	25.87
5: H_sapiens|P09211|p1	26.47	28.99	28.71	20.59	100.00	24.48	19.57	17.72
6: H_sapiens|O60760|s1	24.34	25.26	25.93	21.05	24.48	100.00	19.10	22.78
7: H_sapiens|P30711|t1	16.84	16.32	19.25	18.65	19.57	19.10	100.00	25.28
8: H_sapiens|O43708|z1	16.36	21.76	14.56	25.87	17.72	22.78	25.28	100.00

Figure 1.
Alignment of the amino acid sequences of Ts26GST with representatives of different human GST classes. The percent identity matrix shows that Ts26GST is most related to human M-class GST (m1).

T. solium (see **Table 1**). Furthermore, the kinetic curves for both substrates showed positive cooperativity, indicating that the binding of the first substrate stabilizes the right conformation of Ts26GST to bind the second substrate [21]. This positive cooperativity, previously described for the GSTs of *P. falciparum* and in classes P1 and Z1 of mammals, allows the parasite to adapt to changes in the amounts of toxic molecules secreted by the host's immune cells or induced by oral drugs, and to inactivate them through efficient processing of these substrates [69].

Kinetic analyses performed at different concentrations of GSH and CDNB produced intersecting double-reciprocal plots that provided evidence of ternary complex formation during enzymatic conjugation [70]. Furthermore, because the intersection occurred on the abscissa, the mechanism proceeds through the random sequential binding of co-substrates [71].

To determine the GST class to which Ts26GST belongs, various class marker substrates and inhibitors were tested. Ts26GST conjugates the A-class markers cumene hydroperoxide and ethacrynic acid better than the M-class marker 1,2-dichloro-4-nitrobenzene [20]. However, Ts26GST is more sensitive to the M-class inhibitors cibacron blue and triphenyltin chloride than to bromosulfophtalein, an A-class inhibitor. This enzyme is also sensitive to the anthelminthic mebendazole, displaying a non-competitive inhibition pattern, which suggests that at least two molecules bind to Ts26GST [21].

3.2 Structural similarity of Ts26GST to human cGSTs

Multiple amino acid sequence alignments of Ts26GST with all classes of human cGSTs are shown in **Figure 1**. It can be seen from the percent identity matrix that the primary structure of Ts26GST is closely related to M-class (42% sequence identity) and A-class (27% sequence identity) but is more distant from other human GST classes. The G-site of Ts26GST belongs to class Y, with Y8 being the catalytic residue that activates GSH. This site also has the essential conserved residues for γ-glutamyl binding: P(57), Q(68), and S(69). The last two residues are part of the (Q)SHVIT sequence, which in mammalian GSTs constitutes the consensus motif (Q)SNAIL /(Q)TRAIL. Notably, amino acid variation in this consensus motif is one of the markers for distinguishing between mammalian and

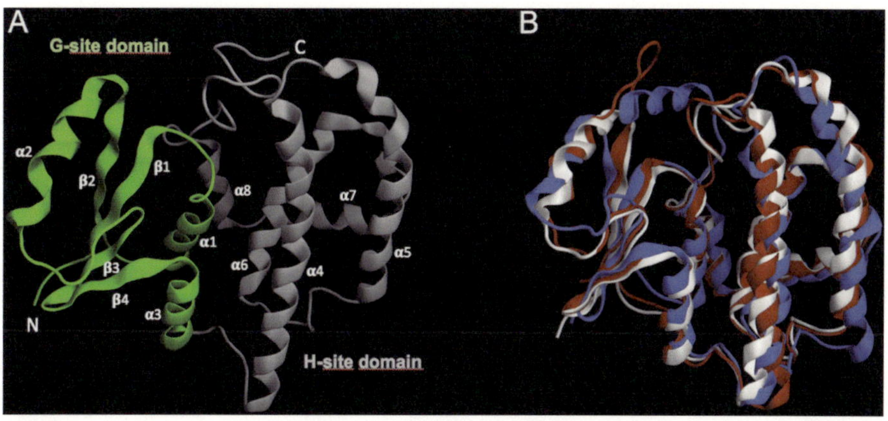

Figure 2.
Modeled structure of Ts26GST. (A) The domain with the site where glutathione binds, is highlighted in green, and the domain with the hydrophobic site, to which electrophilic substrates bind, is highlighted in gray. (B) The structure of Ts26GST in white is compared to human A-class GST structure (blue) and M-class structure (brown).

parasite cGSTs [20]. Ts26GST has ligandin activity and is internalized by macrophages, suggesting an important role in transport and the parasite–host relationship [72, 73].

A homology model for Ts26GST was built from the structure of *Fasciola hepatica* M-class GST (PDB ID 2FHE), whose sequence has 47% identity, with 96% query coverage [70]. The analysis of this model with PROCHECK showed that 91.5% of residues are in favored regions in the Ramachandran plot, with no residues in the disallowed region. In addition, verification with ERRAT yielded an Overall Quality Factor of 93.55 and the Verify3D score was 95.18. A comparison of the Ts26GST model with M and A-class human GST structures is shown in **Figure 2**. It is clear that Ts26GST does not have the classical mammalian mu-loop or the canonical α9-helix observed in A-class GSTs.

4. Structure-based discovery of Ts26GST selective inhibitors

4.1 Search and selection of cavities with non-conserved residues as potential targets

Knowing the structure of the target whose activity we wish to inhibit is an essential step for the discovery and optimization of specific inhibitors. Furthermore, if the target is a parasitic enzyme, and the host has orthologs, knowing and comparing their structures allows us to take advantage of their differences and design more specific inhibitors [74]. Different strategies have been used to find appropriate inhibitors, and we decided to look for a non-competitive inhibitor that cannot be displaced by excess substrate, i.e., the one that would not bind to either the G-site or the H-site. Thus, we focused our search on the area of the dimer interface, trying to find a site whose occupation would alter the architecture of at least one of the substrate sites and prevent catalysis. Furthermore, the binding of a molecule in this interfacial region could destabilize the quaternary structure of this enzyme, which is only active as a dimer. Likewise, we assumed that the site has a predominantly hydrophobic surface and contains a considerable fraction of non-conserved residues with respect to its human orthologs. Using the MOE's Site Finder tool [75], we found only one site that met all these requirements; its location is shown in **Figure 3**.

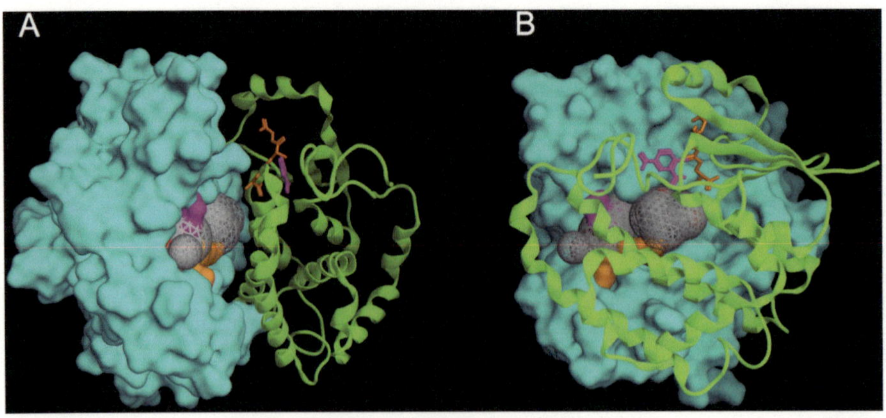

Figure 3.
Putative binding site for TS26GST inhibitors whose occupancy could produce non-competitive inhibition. Just one subunit is represented with van der Waals surface for clarity. Bound GSH and CDNB molecules are shown in orange and magenta, respectively, whereas the spheres represent the space that the ligand could occupy.

4.2 Virtual screening with a commercial diverse library set

Once a potential inhibitor binding site has been located, we must find molecules that conform to its surface and interact favorably to form stable complexes. To explore how to cover this site in the chemical space, we used Enamine's library of non-redundant organic compounds called the Discovery Diversity Set, which consists of 50,240 drug-like compounds, and performed virtual screening using AutoDock Vina [76]. The scores of the best candidates were verified using MOE's Dock Tool [75].

4.3 Assortment of candidates

The best putative binders for Ts26GST were selected using the conventional criteria: the highest docking scores, the highest number of hydrogen bonds, and Lipinski's rule of five [77], but in addition, those ligands were prioritized that established the lowest number of contacts with conserved residues in relation to human GSTs. The best 23 candidates are shown in **Figure 4** and their docking scores obtained using AutoDock Vina and MOE are given in **Table 2**.

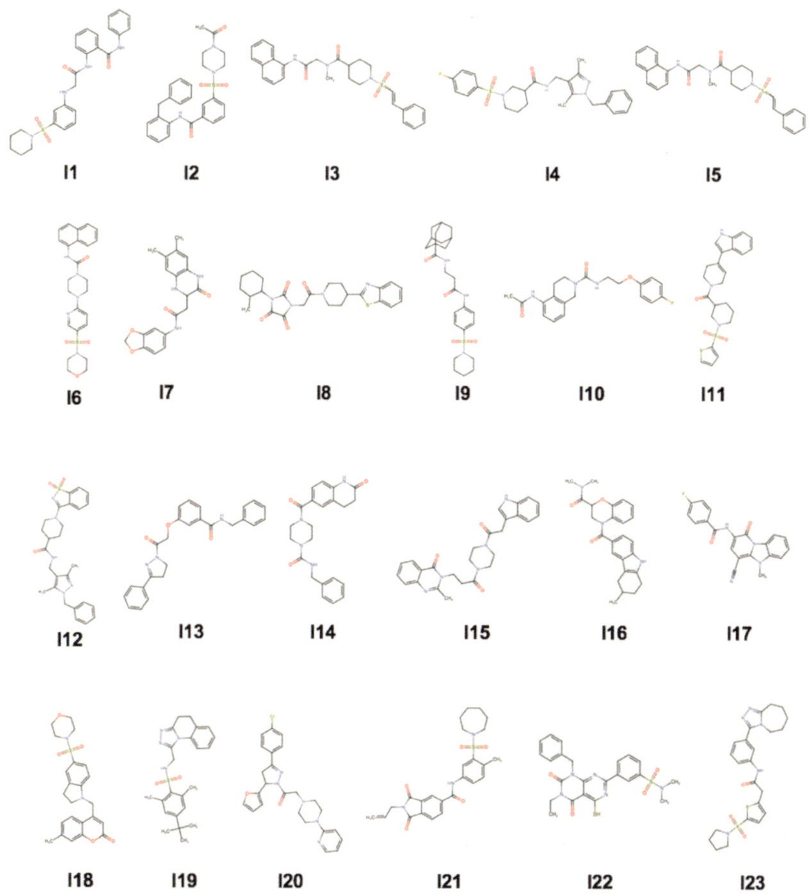

Figure 4.
Best candidate inhibitors found by virtual screening.

Compound	Enamine ID	Chemical formula	Docking score VINA/MOE	*Residual activity (%)
I1	Z30971507	$C_{26}H_{28}N_4O_4S$	−9.6/−11.1	92
I2	Z26762460	$C_{26}H_{27}N_3O_4S$	−10.0/−10.4	129
I3	Z27434387	$C_{22}H_{21}FN_4O_3S_2$	−9.4/−10.1	98
I4	Z109818646	$C_{25}H_{29}FN_4O_3S$	−9.4/−11.0	120
I5	Z27205337	$C_{27}H_{29}N_3O_4S$	−9.5/−10.3	82
I6	Z235256042	$C_{24}H_{27}N_5O_4S$	−10.0/−10.3	74
I7	Z56803795	$C_{19}H_{19}N_3O_4$	−9.9/−9.7	30
I8	Z98069587	$C_{24}H_{28}N_4O_4S$	−9.9/−9.7	107
I9	Z51980171	$C_{25}H_{35}N_3O_4S$	−9.5/−10.8	76
I10	Z744434314	$C_{20}H_{22}FN_3O_3$	−9.4/−10.2	135
I11	Z231257554	$C_{23}H_{25}N_3O_3S_2$	−9.5/−10.0	83
I12	Z109816768	$C_{26}H_{29}N_5O_3S$	−9.9/−9.8	117
I13	Z225448008	$C_{25}H_{23}N_3O_3$	−9.4/−10.1	55
I14	Z283658802	$C_{22}H_{24}N_4O_3$	−9.7/−8.8	115
I15	Z512929356	$C_{26}H_{27}N_5O_3$	−9.8/−9.3	114
I16	Z131580092	$C_{25}H_{27}N_3O_3$	−9.7/−9.9	108
I17	Z90661741	$C_{20}H_{13}FN_4O_2$	−9.8/−8.5	116
I18	Z134793448	$C_{23}H_{24}N_2O_5S$	−9.9/−10.3	66
I19	Z317185036	$C_{23}H_{28}N_4O_2S$	−9.9/−10.0	113
I20	Z30996502	$C_{24}H_{24}ClN_5O_2$	−9.4/−10.6	72
I21	Z26496603	$C_{25}H_{27}N_3O_5S$	−9.9/−11.5	78
I22	Z55180729	$C_{23}H_{23}N_5O_4S_2$	−9.6/−9.9	88
I23	Z30414302	$C_{23}H_{27}N_5O_3S_2$	−9.7/−10.0	82

Residual activity of 5 μg of recombinant Ts26GST in presence of 100 μM of potential inhibitors.

Table 2.
Docking scores of the predicted potential inhibitors determined using Vina and MOE_Dock. The inhibitory capacity of the compounds was determined by measuring the enzymatic activity of T26GST in the presence of each compound at a concentration of 100 μM, with 5.0 mM GSH and 2.5 mM CDNB. The reaction rate was monitored by ultraviolet–visible absorption at 340 nm and compared with that obtained in the absence of the compound (100% activity).

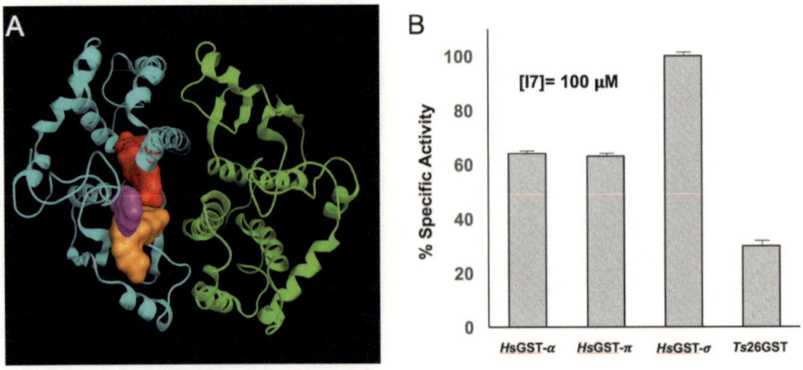

Figure 5.
Relative position of the substrates GSH (orange) and CDNB (magenta), and the inhibitor I7 (red) in the structure of Ts26GST. (A) This figure was obtained by the superposition of the crystallographic structures of the complex M-class GS-DNB-HsGST (PDB ID: 1XWK) with the modeled complex of Ts26GST-I7, hiding the protein chain of the human GST. (B) Percent residual activity of Ts26GST and three human GSTs in the presence of 100 μM I7.

4.4 *In vitro* assay of selected compounds with the best scores

The twenty-three compounds previously identified as potential ligands of Ts26GST were purchased and tested for their inhibitory activity using *in vitro* enzymatic assays. **Table 2** shows the residual activity obtained with 5.0 μg of recombinant Ts26GST in the presence of each compound at a concentration of 100 μM. I7 was the best Enamine compound that inhibited enzymatic activity of Ts26GST by 70%. **Figure 5A** shows the location of the I7 binding site, as derived from the docking protocol. We also tested the inhibitory effect of I7 on several human GSTs and observed that it had much smaller or no effect (**Figure 5B**).

5. Conclusions

Human NCC caused by *T. solium* larvae can be asymptomatic, disabling, and sometimes fatal. Currently, its diagnosis and treatment are expensive, and the approved drugs have associated unwanted effects. The search for the essential targets in *T. solium*, such as GST, and the methodology used to obtain the inhibitor I7 and its derivatives, shows that it is possible to develop safe, specific, and effective drugs that will contribute to eradicating this parasite. We are currently working on the crystallization of Ts26GST and site-directed mutagenesis to verify the location of the I7 binding site.

Acknowledgements

This work was supported by National Council of Science and Technology of Mexico (National Problems CONACYTPN-594) and (Frontier Science 2019 (7397); General Direction of Academic Staff Affairs at the National Autonomous University of Mexico (DGAPA-PAPIIT-IN217419), and the Direction of Computing and Technologies of Information and Communication (Miztli-LANCAD-UNAM-DGTIC-344). The authors thank the facilities provided by the Supercomputing and Parallel Visualization Laboratory at the Metropolitan Autonomous University, Iztapalapa Campus.

Conflict of interest

The authors declare that they have no known conflict of interest.

Author details

Rafael A. Zubillaga[1], Lucía Jiménez[2], Ponciano García-Gutiérrez[1] and Abraham Landa[2*]

1 Department of Chemistry, Metropolitan Autonomous University, Mexico City, Mexico

2 Department of Microbiology and Parasitology, Faculty of Medicine, National Autonomous University of Mexico, Mexico City, Mexico

*Address all correspondence to: landap@unam.mx

References

[1] Fleury A, Escobar A, Fragoso G, Sciutto E, Larralde C. Clinical heterogeneity of human neurocysticercosis results from complex interactions among parasite, host and environmental factors. Trans R Soc Trop Med Hyg. 2010;104:243-250. doi: 10.1016/j.trstmh.2010.01.005

[2] Garcia HH, Nash TE, Del Brutto OH. Clinical symptoms, diagnosis, and treatment of neurocysticercosis. Lancet Neurol. 2014;13:1202-15. doi: 10.1016/S1474-4422(14)70094-8

[3] Carabin H, Ndimubanzi PC, Budke CM, Nguyen H, Qian Y, Cowan LD, Stoner JA, Rainwater E, Dickey M. Clinical manifestations associated with neurocysticercosis: a systematic review. PLoS Negl Trop Dis. 2011;5:e1152. doi: 10.1371/journal.pntd.0001152

[4] Sotelo J. Clinical manifestations, diagnosis, and treatment of neurocysticercosis. Curr Neurol Neurosci Rep. 2011;11:529-35. doi: 10.1007/s11910-011-0226-7

[5] Del Brutto OH. Neurocysticercosis. Neurohospitalist. 2014;4:205-12. doi: 10.1177/1941874414533351.

[6] Madrazo I, García-Rentería JA, Sandoval M, López Vega FJ. Intraventricular cysticercosis. Neurosurgery. 1983;12:148-52. doi: 10.1227/00006123-198302000-00003

[7] Sinha S, Sharma BS. Intraventricular neurocysticercosis: a review of current status and management issues. Br J Neurosurg. 2012;26:305-9. doi: 10.3109/02688697.2011.635820. Epub 2011 Dec 15

[8] Bhattarai R, Carabin H, Proaño JV, Flores-Rivera J, Corona T, Flisser A, León-Maldonado L, Budke CM. The monetary burden of cysticercosis in Mexico. PLoS Negl Trop Dis. 2019;13(7):e0007501. doi: 10.1371/journal.pntd.0007501

[9] Rajkotia Y, Lescano AG, Gilman RH, Cornejo C, Garcia HH; Cysticercosis Working Group of Peru. Economic burden of neurocysticercosis: results from Peru. Trans R Soc Trop Med Hyg. 2007;101:840-6. doi: 10.1016/j.trstmh.2007.03.008

[10] García HH, Evans CA, Nash TE, Takayanagui OM, White AC Jr, Botero D, Rajshekhar V, Tsang VC, Schantz PM, Allan JC, Flisser A, Correa D, Sarti E, Friedland JS, Martinez SM, Gonzalez AE, Gilman RH, Del Brutto OH. Current consensus guidelines for treatment of neurocysticercosis. Clin Microbiol Rev. 2002;15:747-56. doi: 10.1128/cmr.15.4.747-756.2002

[11] Overbosch D, van de Nes JC, Groll E, Diekmann HW, Polderman AM, Mattie H. Penetration of praziquantel into cerebrospinal fluid and cysticerci in human cysticercosis. Eur J Clin Pharmacol. 1987;33:287-92. doi: 10.1007/BF00637564

[12] Sotelo J, Jung H. Pharmacokinetic optimisation of the treatment of neurocysticercosis. Clin Pharmacokinet. 1998;34:503-15. doi: 10.2165/00003088-199834060-00006

[13] White AC Jr, Garcia HH. Updates on the management of neurocysticercosis. Curr Opin Infect Dis. 2018;31:377-382. doi: 10.1097/QCO.0000000000000480

[14] Lacey E. Mode of action of benzimidazoles. Parasitol Today. 1990;6:112-5. doi: 10.1016/0169-4758(90)90227-u. PMID: 15463312

[15] Jung H, Hurtado M, Sanchez M, Medina MT, Sotelo J. Plasma and CSF levels of albendazole and praziquantel

in patients with neurocysticercosis. Clin Neuropharmacol. 1990;13:559-64. doi: 10.1097/00002826-199012000-00008

[16] Gonzalez AE, Bustos JA, Jimenez JA, Rodriguez ML, Ramirez MG, Gilman RH, Garcia HH; Cysticercosis Working Group in Peru. Efficacy of diverse antiparasitic treatments for cysticercosis in the pig model. Am J Trop Med Hyg. 2012;87:292-6. doi: 10.4269/ajtmh.2012.11-0371

[17] Cohen L, Belec L, Sanson M, Pierrot-Deseilligny C, Signoret JL: Selective sensitivity of cysts to praziquantel and albendazole in a case of cerebral cysticercosis. Rev Neurol. 1992,148:58-61.

[18] Cárdenas, G., Carrillo-Mezo, R., Jung, H., Sciutto, E., Hernandez, J. L., Fleury, A. Subarachnoidal Neurocysticercosis non-responsive to cysticidal drugs: a case series. BMC neurology, 2010;10, 16. https://doi.org/10.1186/1471-2377-10-16

[19] Vibanco-Pérez, N., Jiménez, L., Mendoza-Hernández, G., Landa, A. Characterization of a recombinant mu-class glutathione S-transferase from Taenia solium. Parasitol. Res. 2002;88:398-404. doi: 10.1007/s00436-001-0580-5

[20] Torres-Rivera A, Landa A. Glutathione transferases from parasites: a biochemical view. Acta Trop. 2008a;105(2):99-112. doi: 10.1016/j.actatropica.2007.08.005

[21] Torres-Rivera A, Landa A. Cooperative kinetics of the recombinant glutathione transferase of Taenia solium and characterization of the enzyme. Arch Biochem Biophys. 2008b;477:372-8. doi: 10.1016/j.abb.2008.07.008. Epub 2008 Jul 17

[22] Tsai IJ, Zarowiecki M, Holroyd N, Garciarrubio A, Sánchez-Flores A, Brooks KL, Tracey A, Bobes RJ, Fragoso G, Sciutto E, Aslett M, Beasley H, Bennett HM, Cai X, Camicia F, Clark R, Cucher M, De Silva N, Day TA, Deplazes P, Estrada K, Fernández C, Holland PWH, Hou J, Hu S, Huckvale T, Hung SS, Kamenetzky L, Keane JA, Kiss F, Koziol U, Lambert O, Liu K, Luo X, Luo Y, Macchiaroli N, Nichol S, Paps J, Parkinson J, Pouchkina-Stantcheva N, Riddiford N, Rosenzvit M, Salinas G, Wasmuth JD, Zamanian M, Zheng Y; Taenia solium Genome Consortium, Cai J, Soberón X, Olson PD, Laclette JP, Brehm K, Berriman M. The genomes of four tapeworm species reveal adaptations to parasitism. Nature. 2013;496:57-63. doi: 10.1038/nature12031. Epub 2013 Mar 13

[23] Brophy PM, Pritchard DI. Parasitic helminth glutathione S-transferases: an update on their potential as targets for immuno- and chemotherapy. Exp Parasitol. 1994;79:89-96. doi: 10.1006/expr.1994.1067

[24] Tew KD, Dutta S, Schultz M. Inhibitors of glutathione S-transferases as therapeutic agents. Adv Drug Deliv Rev. 1997;26:91-104. doi: 10.1016/s0169-409x(97)00029-x

[25] Armstrong RN. Structure, catalytic mechanism, and evolution of the glutathione transferases. Chem Res Toxicol. 1997;10:2-18. doi: 10.1021/tx960072x

[26] Suzuki T, Nishio K, Tanabe S. The MRP family and anticancer drug metabolism. Curr Drug Metab. 2001;2:367-77. doi: 10.2174/1389200013338289

[27] Clark AG. The comparative enzymology of the glutathione S-transferases from non-vertebrate organisms. Comp Biochem Physiol B. 1989;92(3):419-46. doi: 10.1016/0305-0491(89)90114-4.

[28] Van Bladeren PJ. Glutathione conjugation as a bioactivation reaction.

Chem Biol Interact. 2000;129:61-76. doi: 10.1016/s0009-2797(00)00214-3

[29] Wilce MC, Parker MW. Structure and function of glutathione S-transferases. Biochim Biophys Acta. 1994;1205:1-18. doi: 10.1016/0167-4838(94)90086-8

[30] Mannervik B, Board PG, Hayes JD, Listowsky I, Pearson WR. Nomenclature for mammalian soluble glutathione transferases. Methods Enzymol. 2005;401:1-8. doi: 10.1016/S0076-6879(05)01001-3

[31] Frova C. Glutathione transferases in the genomics era: new insights and perspectives. Biomol Eng. 2006;23:149-69. doi: 10.1016/j.bioeng.2006.05.020

[32] Morel F, Aninat C. The glutathione transferase kappa family. Drug Metab Rev. 2011;43:281-91. doi: 10.3109/03602532.2011.556122

[33] Hayes JD, Flanagan JU, Jowsey IR. Glutathione transferases. Annu Rev Pharmacol Toxicol. 2005; 45:51-88. doi: 10.1146/annurev.pharmtox.45.120403.095857

[34] Oakley AJ. Glutathione transferases: new functions. Curr Opin Struct Biol. 2005;15:716-23. doi: 10.1016/j.sbi.2005.10.005.

[35] Jakobsson PJ, Morgenstern R, Mancini J, Ford-Hutchinson A, Persson B. Common structural features of MAPEG--a widespread superfamily of membrane associated proteins with highly divergent functions in eicosanoid and glutathione metabolism. Protein Sci. 1999;8:689-92. doi: 10.1110/ps.8.3.689

[36] Jakobsson PJ, Morgenstern R, Mancini J, Ford-Hutchinson A, Persson B. Membrane-associated proteins in eicosanoid and glutathione metabolism (MAPEG). A widespread protein superfamily. Am J Respir Crit Care Med. 2000;161:S20-4. doi: 10.1164/ajrccm.161.supplement_1.ltta-5.

[37] Bresell A, Weinander R, Lundqvist G, Raza H, Shimoji M, Sun TH, Balk L, Wiklund R, Eriksson J, Jansson C, Persson B, Jakobsson PJ, Morgenstern R. Bioinformatic and enzymatic characterization of the MAPEG superfamily. FEBS J. 2005;272:1688-703. doi: 10.1111/j.1742-4658.2005.04596.x

[38] Board PG, Coggan M, Watson S, Gage PW, Dulhunty AF. CLIC-2 modulates cardiac ryanodine receptor Ca2+ release channels. Int J Biochem Cell Biol. 2004;36:1599-612. doi: 10.1016/j.biocel.2004.01.026

[39] Cho, S.G., Lee, Y.H., Park, H.S., Ryoo, K., Kank, K.W., Park, J., Eom, S.J., Kim, M.J., Chang, T.S., Choi, S.Y., Shim, J., Kim, Y., Dong, M.J., Kim, S.G., Ichijo, H., Choi, F.J. Glutathione S-transferase mu modulates the stress-activated signals by suppressing apoptosis signal-regulating kinase 1. J. Biol. Chem. 2001;276:12749-12755. doi: 10.1074/jbc.M005561200.

[40] Herve, M. Pivotal roles of the parasite PGD2 synthase and of the host D prostanoid receptor 1 in schistosome immune evasion. Eur. J. Immunol. 2003;33:2764-2772.

[41] Ketterer B. Detoxication reactions of glutathione and glutathione transferases. Xenobiotica. 1986;16:957-73. doi: 10.3109/00498258609038976.

[42] Mannervik B. The isoenzymes of glutathione transferase. Adv Enzymol Relat Areas Mol Biol. 1985; 57:357-417. doi: 10.1002/9780470123034.ch5

[43] Tsuchida S, Izumi T, Shimizu T, Ishikawa T, Hatayama I, Satoh K, Sato K. Purification of a new acidic glutathione S-transferase, GST-Yn1Yn1, with a high leukotriene-C4 synthase activity from rat brain. Eur J Biochem.

1987;170:159-64. doi: 10.1111/j.1432-1033.1987.tb13681.x

[44] Eaton DL, Bammler TK. Concise review of the glutathione S-transferases and their significance to toxicology. Toxicol Sci. 1999;49:156-64. doi: 10.1093/toxsci/49.2.156

[45] Sheehan D, Meade G, Foley VM, Dowd CA. Structure, function and evolution of glutathione transferases: implications for classification of non-mammalian members of an ancient enzyme superfamily. Biochem J. 2001;360:1-16. doi: 10.1042/0264-6021:3600001

[46] Ishikawa T, Li ZS, Lu YP, Rea PA. The GS-X pump in plant, yeast, and animal cells: structure, function, and gene expression. Biosci Rep. 1997;17:189-207. doi: 10.1023/a:1027385513483

[47] Ishikawa T. The ATP-dependent glutathione S-conjugate export pump. Trends Biochem Sci. 1992;17:463-8. doi: 10.1016/0968-0004(92)90489-v

[48] Dirr HW, Wallace LA. Role of the C-terminal helix 9 in the stability and ligandin function of class alpha glutathione transferase A1-1. Biochemistry. 1999;38:15631-40. doi: 10.1021/bi991179x. PMID: 10569948

[49] Allocati N, Masulli M, Di Ilio C, Federici L. Glutathione transferases: substrates, inihibitors and pro-drugs in cancer and neurodegenerative diseases. Oncogenesis. 2018;7:8. doi: 10.1038/s41389-017-0025-3

[50] Ji X, von Rosenvinge EC, Johnson WW, Armstrong RN, Gilliland GL. Location of a potential transport binding site in a sigma class glutathione transferase by x-ray crystallography. Proc Natl Acad Sci U S A. 1996;93(16):8208-13. doi: 10.1073/pnas.93.16.8208

[51] Ketley JN, Habig WH, Jakoby WB. Binding of nonsubstrate ligands to the glutathione S-transferases. J Biol Chem. 1975;250:8670-3

[52] Litwack G, Ketterer B, Arias IM. Ligandin: a hepatic protein which binds steroids, bilirubin, carcinogens and a number of exogenous organic anions. Nature. 1971;234:466-7. doi: 10.1038/234466a0

[53] Morris MJ, Craig SJ, Sutherland TM, Board PG, Casarotto MG. Transport of glutathione transferase-fold structured proteins into living cells. Biochim Biophys Acta. 2009;1788:676-85. doi: 10.1016/j.bbamem.2008.10.018

[54] Namiki S, Tomida T, Tanabe M, Iino M, Hirose K. Intracellular delivery of glutathione S-transferase into mammalian cells. Biochem Biophys Res Commun. 2003;305:592-7. doi: 10.1016/s0006-291x(03)00807-6

[55] Lopez-Gonzalez V, La-Rocca S, Arbildi P, Fernandez V. Characterization of catalytic and non-catalytic activities of EgGST2-3, a heterodimeric glutathione transferase from Echinococcus granulosus. Acta Trop. 2018180:69-75. doi: 10.1016/j.actatropica.2018.01.007

[56] Vibanco-Pérez N, Landa-Piedra A. Glutathione S-transferase in helminth parasites. Rev Latinoam Microbiol. 1998;40:73-85.

[57] Capron A, Riveau G, Grzych JM, Boulanger D, Capron M, Pierce R. Development of a vaccine strategy against human and bovine schistosomiasis. Background and update. Trop Geogr Med. 1994;46:242-6.

[58] Sexton JL, Milner AR, Panaccio M, Waddington J, Wijffels G, Chandler D, Thompson C, Wilson L, Spithill TW, Mitchell GF, et al. Glutathione S-transferase. Novel vaccine against

Fasciola hepatica infection in sheep. J Immunol. 1990;145(11):3905-10

[59] Riveau G, Poulain-Godefroy OP, Dupré L, Remoué F, Mielcarek N, Locht C, Capron A. Glutathione S-transferases of 28kDa as major vaccine candidates against schistosomiasis. Mem Inst Oswaldo Cruz. 1998;93 Suppl 1:87-94. doi: 10.1590/s0074-02761998000700012

[60] Capron A, Riveau G, Capron M, Trottein F. Schistosomes: the road from host-parasite interactions to vaccines in clinical trials. Trends Parasitol. 2005;21:143-9. doi: 10.1016/j.pt.2005.01.003.

[61] Cheng PC, Lin CN, Peng SY, Kang TF, Lee KM. Combined IL-12 Plasmid and Recombinant SjGST Enhance the Protective and Anti-pathology Effect of SjGST DNA Vaccine Against Schistosoma japonicum. PLoS Negl Trop Dis. 2016;10:e0004459. doi: 10.1371/journal.pntd.0004459.

[62] Mbanefo EC, Kumagai T, Kodama Y, Kurosaki T, Furushima-Shimogawara R, Cherif MS, Mizukami S, Kikuchi M, Huy NT, Ohta N, Sasaki H, Hirayama K. Immunogenicity and anti-fecundity effect of nanoparticle coated glutathione S-transferase (SjGST) DNA vaccine against murine Schistosoma japonicum infection. Parasitol Int. 2015;64:24-31. doi: 10.1016/j.parint.2015.01.005

[63] Nava G, Robert L, Plancarte A. Characterization of Taenia solium cysticerci microsomal glutathione S-transferase activity. Parasitol Res. 2007;101:1373-81. doi: 10.1007/s00436-007-0655-z.

[64] Nguyen HA, Bae YA, Lee EG, Kim SH, Diaz-Camacho SP, Nawa Y, Kang I, Kong Y. A novel sigma-like glutathione transferase of Taenia solium metacestode. Int J Parasitol. 2010;40:1097-106. doi: 10.1016/j.ijpara.2010.03.007

[65] Mandour ME, el Turabi H, Homeida MM, el Sadig T, Ali HM, Bennett JL, Leahey WJ, Harron DW. Pharmacokinetics of praziquantel in healthy volunteers and patients with schistosomiasis. Trans R Soc Trop Med Hyg. 1990;84:389-93. doi: 10.1016/0035-9203(90)90333-a

[66] Ridtitid W, Ratsamemonthon K, Mahatthanatrakul W, Wongnawa M. Pharmacokinetic interaction between ketoconazole and praziquantel in healthy volunteers. J Clin Pharm Ther. 2007;32:585-93. doi: 10.1111/j.1365-2710.2007.00862.x

[67] Morgan AS, Ciaccio PJ, Tew KD, Kauvar LM. Isozyme-specific glutathione S-transferase inhibitors potentiate drug sensitivity in cultured human tumor cell lines. Cancer Chemother Pharmacol. 1996;37:363-70. doi: 10.1007/s002800050398

[68] Van Iersel ML, Ploemen JP, Lo Bello M, Federici G, van Bladeren PJ. Interactions of alpha, beta-unsaturated aldehydes and ketones with human glutathione S-transferase P1-1. Chem Biol Interact. 1997;108:67-78. doi: 10.1016/s0009-2797(97)00096-3

[69] Ricci, G., Turella, P., De Maria, F., Antonini, G., Nardocci, L., Board, P.G., Parker, M.W., Carbonelli, M.G., Federici, G., Caccuria, A.M. Binding and kinetic mechanisms of the zeta class glutathione transferase. J. Biol. Chem. 2004;279:33336-33342. doi: 10.1074/jbc.M404631200

[70] García-Gutiérrez P, Zubillaga RA, Téllez-Plancarte A, Flores-López R, Camarillo-Cadena M, Landa A. Discovery of a new non-substrate inhibitor of the 26.5 kDa glutathione transferase from Taenia solium by virtual screening. J Mol Graph Model.

2020;100:107707. doi: 10.1016/j.jmgm.2020.107707

[71] Stefanidis L, Scinto KV, Strada MI, Alper BJ. Bisubstrate kinetics of glutathione S-transferase: a colorimetric experiment for the introductory biochemistry laboratory. J Chem Edu. 2018;95:146-151. doi: 10.1021/acs.jchemed.7b00535

[72] Plancarte A, Romero JR, Nava G, Reyes H, Hernández M. Evaluation of the non-catalytic binding function of Ts26GST a glutathione transferase isoform of Taenia solium. Exp Parasitol. 2014;138:63-70. doi: 10.1016/j.exppara.2014.02.004

[73] Vega-Angeles VT, Terrazas LI, Ledesma-Soto Y, Jiménez L, Landa A. Taenia solium glutathione transferase fraction activates macrophages and favors the development of Th1-type response. Biosci Rep. 2019;39(1):BSR20181132. doi: 10.1042/BSR20181132

[74] Gómez-Puyou A, Saavedra-Lira E, Becker I, Zubillaga RA, Rojo-Domínguez A, Pérez-Montfort R. Using evolutionary changes to achieve species-specific inhibition of enzyme action – studies with triosephosphate isomerase. Chem Biol. 1995;2:847-855. doi: 10.1016/1074-5521(95)90091-8

[75] Molecular Operating Environment (MOE). Chemical Computing Group. Montreal, QC, Canada. 2015. Available from: https://www.chemcomp.com

[76] Trott O, Olson AJ. AutoDock Vina: improving the speed and accuracy of docking with a new scoring function, efficient optimization, and multithreading. J Comput Chem 2010;31:455-461. doi: 10.1002/jcc.21334

[77] Lipinski CA, Lombardo F, Dominy BW, Feeney PJ. Experimental and computational approaches to estimate solubility and permeability in drug discovery and development setting. Adv Drug Deliv Rev. 2001;46:3-26. doi: 10.1016/s0169-409x(00)00129-0

Section 4

The Host-Parasite Interaction

Chapter 7

To Be or Not to Be a Tapeworm Parasite: That Is the Post-Genomic Question in *Taenia solium* Cysticercosis

Diana G. Ríos-Valencia, José Navarrete-Perea, Arturo Calderón-Gallegos, Jeannette Flores-Bautista and Juan Pedro Laclette

Abstract

Cestode parasites rely on their host to obtain their nutrients. Elucidation of tapeworm genomes has shown a remarkable reduction in the coding of multiple enzymes, particularly those of anabolic pathways. Previous findings showed that 10–13% of the proteins found in the vesicular fluid of *Taenia solium* cysticerci are of host origin. Further proteomic characterization allowed identification of 4,259 different proteins including 891 of host origin in the parasite's protein lysates. One explanation for this high abundance and diversity of host proteins in the parasite lysates is related to the functional exploitation of host proteins by cysticerci. Supporting this concept is the uptake of host haptoglobin and hemoglobin by the parasite, as a way to acquire iron. Surprisingly, internalized host proteins are minimally degraded by the parasite physiological machinery. Additional proteomic analysis demonstrated that these host proteins become part of the organic matrix of calcareous corpuscles; as 60–70% of the protein content are host proteins. In this review, a collection of available genomic and proteomic data for taeniid cestodes is assembled, the subject of the use and processing of host proteins is particularly addressed; a sketchy and unique cell physiological profile starts to emerge for these parasitic organisms.

Keywords: *Taenia solium*, Cestoda, Genome, Proteome, Host proteins, Calcareous Corpuscles

1. Introduction

Tapeworms are invertebrate metazoans producing zoonotic parasite diseases in animals and humans. These parasites have a worldwide distribution, but they especially affect human populations in developing countries and are considered neglected diseases [1]. Their larvae, known as metacestodes (including forms such as cysticercus in *Taenia solium* or hydatid or alveolar cysts in *Echinococcus* sp.) cause the highest morbidities due to tapeworms [2, 3], since they can produce generalized organ failure or seizures and can even result in patient's death [4–7].

Tapeworms produce long-term infections, being able to survive within its host for several years [8], maintaining a dynamic and complex host-parasite relationship [9]. Their lifecycles involve two host (intermediate and final) and include several developmental stages: embryo, larvae and adult stage [10] that can lodge in different tissues of their hosts producing diseases with a wide range of clinical presentations [11].

After description of the genomes of four tapeworms in 2013 [12], molecular studies of these organism have entered an integrative era; including approaches involving genomics, transcriptomics and proteomics [13]. These approaches are presented as promising avenues for the discovery of new pathways to improve our understanding of parasite diseases caused by cestodes, in the hope of developing better surveillance, treatment and control guidelines.

This chapter reviews current perspectives in the study of flatworms; special emphasis is placed on the genomics and proteomics of cestodes and taeniid parasites. The conspicuous and abundant presence of host proteins is particularly considered for taeniid larval forms.

2. The Platyhelminth genome

Access to massive sequencing technologies allowed characterization of entire genomes for some of the most relevant flatworms; being the free living *Schmidtea mediterranea* the first trematode to be reported in 2008 [14]. The timeline of all flatworms genome projects that have been published to date clearly shows the advent of the post-genomic era of flatworms (**Table 1**). A rapid characterization of the genomes of parasites with medical importance, such as *Schistosoma japonicum, S. mansoni, Clonorchis sinensis*, among others, followed by four cestodes: *Hymenolepis microstoma, Echinococcus granulosus, E. multilocularis and Taenia solium* [12]. Subsequently, the International Helminth Genomes Consortium carried out a project with a goal of 50 helminth genomes. These genomes are currently deposited in the WormBase Parasite database, where users can access 197 genomes [15], including 44 Platyhelminthes: 4 free-living flatworms, 20 trematodes, 19 cestodes and 2 monogeneans (**Figure 1**). This platform also allows searching protein domains and Gene Ontology terms,

	Genome size (Mb)	No. of Genes	Longest scaffold size (Mb)	N50 length (Mb)	N90 length (kb)	GC content (%)
T. solium	122.3	12490	0.7	0.07	5.3	43
T. multiceps	240	12890	10.5	44.8	8500	43.7
T. saginata	169	13,161	7.3	0.58	29.4	43.2
T. asiatica	168	13,323	4.2	0.34	14.3	43.1
E. multilocularis	115	10345	20.1	13.8	2900	42.2
E. granulosus	114.9	10231	16	5.2	200	42
E. canadensis	115	11449	0.574	0.075	3.8	42
E. oligarthrus	86	8756	16	10.2	11.6	41
H. microstoma	141.1	10241	2.4	0.5	82	35.9
H. diminuta	177	15169	6.9	2.3	412.2	35.3

Table 1.
Statistics of completed genome sequencing for several tapeworms.

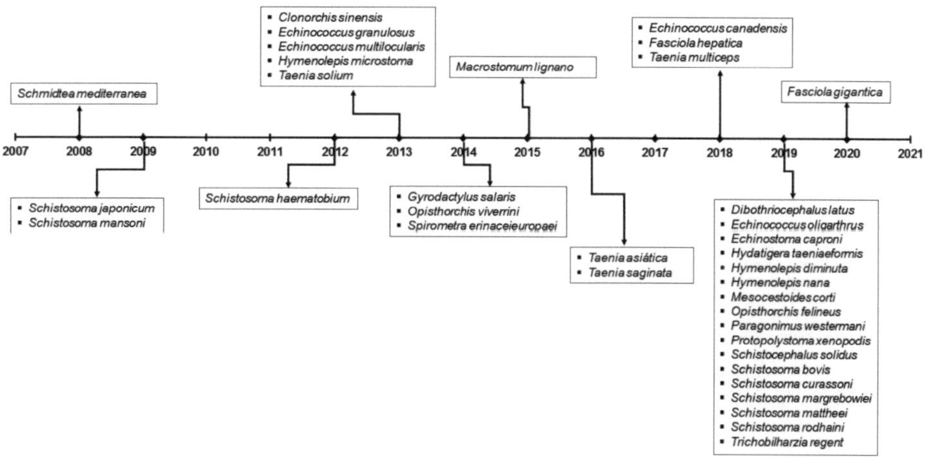

Figure 1.
Timeline of flatworms genome characterization [12, 14–39].

as well as performing comparative analysis of genes and alignments of RNA-Seq data sets, specific to the life stage genomes, among other useful functions [40, 41].

Other taeniid genomes have been reported outside the International Helminth Genomes Consortium during the past five years: *T. asiatica*, *T. saginata* [31] and *T. multiceps* [34], *E. canadensis* [32], *E. oligarthrus* [35], as well as *Hymenolepis diminuta* [36]; circumstances appear prone to greatly improve our understanding of the biology and evolution in those organisms, as well as to solve old unanswered questions on their host-parasite relationships. Availability of this genomic information allows integrative studies on this ancient lineage of organisms. **Table 1** includes the basic statistics of reported assemblies for several tapeworms of medical or veterinary importance, being *E. oligarthrus* the smallest assembly (86 Mb) and *T. multiceps* the largest one (240 Mb). The average GC content of these genomes is 35-43.7%, similar to trematode genomes [23] but different to bacterial genomes whose GC range content is 13.5%-74.9% [42]. As a reference, GC average content of vertebrates is 46% [43]; mice 41.7% [44] whereas human genome is 40.9% [45].

3. Gene gain/reduction along tapeworm evolution

The genomic data of the first four tapeworm genomes sequenced [12] permitted identification of reduction events for groups of genes such as Wnt, which corroborated some data that suggested the loss of these genes in trematodes [46]. Moreover, other genes as Nek kinases, peroxisomal genes and ParaHox members, as well as neuropeptides and G-protein coupled receptors (GPCRs) [15].

The loss of approximately 10 Hox gene families in tapeworms during their evolutionary pathway apparently affected the morphology of those organisms, i.e., the lack of eye-cups and gut [12]; Hox genes such as pax3/7, gbx, hbn and rax are mainly involved in neuronal development or eye development [47–50], as well as ParaHox genes in the formation of the digestive tract [51]. Another type of proteins absent in cestodes are those related to germ cells such as piwi, tudor and Vasa, although the latter have been found possible orthologues in the PL10 family [12].

Tapeworms have developed a specialized detoxification system that includes a single cytochrome p450 gene [12, 52], as well as a redox homeostatic system based on thioredoxin glutathione reductase and the expansion of glutathione

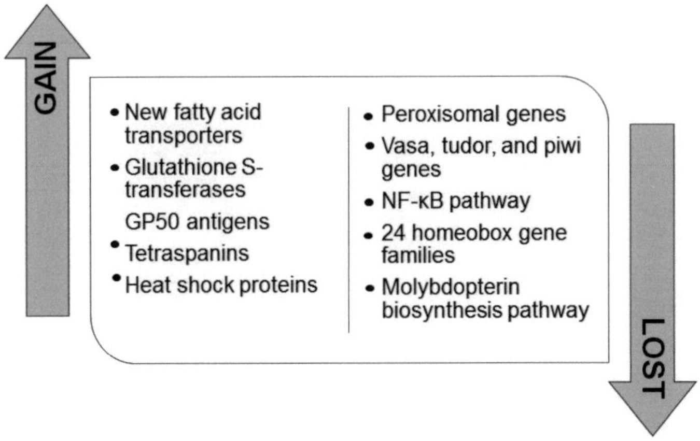

Figure 2.
Gains and losses of genes in taeniids. Phylogenetic study carried out with the genomes of the cestodes allowed finding important aspects about how these organisms acquired or lost some of their genomic traits to adapt to the conditions of their current environments.

S-transferases [53–55]. In addition, there was an expansion of some very specific protein families such as non-canonical heat shock proteins, with *Echinococcus* and *T. solium* having the highest number of genetic expansions in the cytosolic clade Hsp70 [12] suggesting that tapeworms have different mechanisms from nematodes to overcome stress [16]. In addition, taeniids have an expansion in some families of antigens such as GP50 [12, 15]. These antigens are useful for diagnostics; for example, coenurosis in goats [56] or cysticercosis in pigs [57]. For diagnosis of human cysticercosis, the use of GP50 as a diagnostic target allows a 100% specificity and 90% sensitivity using serum samples of patients [58, 59]. Some of the main gains and losses of genes in taeniids are summarized in **Figure 2**.

Our current knowledge on cestode's and taeniid's genomes is still limited but the speed of genomic data acquisition can advance significantly in this new era. We envisage a better understanding of these host–parasite interactions, at a molecular/evolutionary level that can help us unravel events that have permitted the adaptations of these platyhelminths to the host environment.

4. Metabolic adaptations of tapeworms

A great impact of having available complete tapeworm genomes is the characterization of the metabolic pathways in these organisms. Now we know that taeniid tapeworms cannot synthesize fatty acids and cholesterol de novo [25, 60]. For example, KEGG analysis for fatty acid biosynthesis in *T. solium* clearly shows that most of the components of the pathway are absent (**Figure 3**). Therefore, these parasites cannot carry out biosynthesis of fatty acids and are obligated to acquire host fatty acids through specific transporters [63]. Moreover, no genes related to the β-oxidation pathway were found in *Echinococcus* and *Hymenolepis,* although experimental data suggest that other flatworms do carry out this metabolic process [64] for utilization of lipids as a source of energy. It is clear that their major energy source are carbohydrates such as glucose and glycogen. This is supported by the fact that most enzymes participating in carbohydrate catabolism are expressed.

The synthesis of pyrimidines is also absent for taeniids [65], indicating that they acquire pyrimidines from their hosts. The biosynthesis of purines shows a similar landscape [15]. Parasitic flatworms are considered auxotrophic for eight

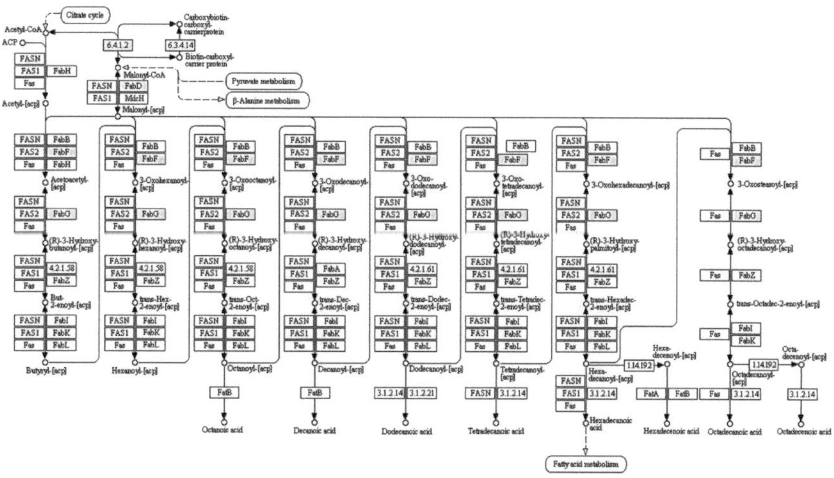

Figure 3.
KEGG analysis of the fatty acid biosynthesis in T. solium*. Enzymes available for this pathway are acetyl-CoA carboxylase (6.4.1.2), S-malonyltranferase (FabF), 3-Oxoacyl-[acyl-carrier-protein] synthetase II (FabF) and Ketoacyl-acyl carrier protein (FabG) [green squares] [61, 62].*

of the nine amino acids that are essential for humans (Phe, His, Lys, Leu, Met, Thr, Trp, and Val). Cestodes have a limited ability to synthesize amino acids, as an example, serine and proline are absent in *E. multilocularis* [16]; biosynthesis of lysine and the aromatic amino acids (Phe, Trp and Tyr) are also absent in most cestodes (**Figure 4**). Arginine is also an essential amino acid in helminths including flatworms, as they do not have all the necessary enzymes of the urea cycle to process

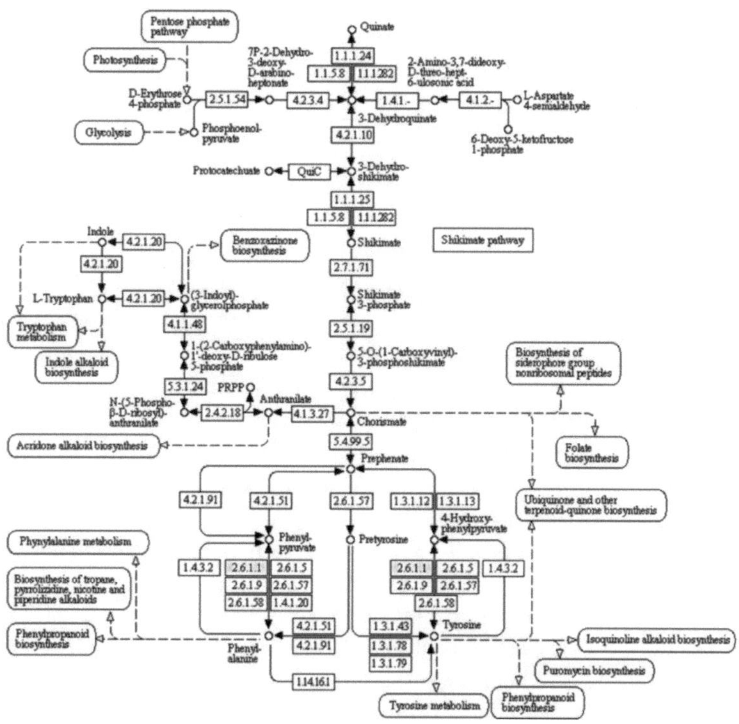

Figure 4.
KEGG analysis of phenylalanine, tyrosine and tryptophan biosynthesis in T. solium*. The only enzymes that are present in the* T. solium *genome are indicated in green within boxes [61, 62].*

ornithine, which is the precursor of arginine [15]. In summary, these parasitic organisms rely on their host for the acquisition of fatty acids, nucleosides and most amino acids. Metabolically speaking, they show highly simplified genomes.

5. Taeniid larval tissues contain large amounts of host proteins

The presence of host proteins in the tissues of the cystic larval forms of taeniids has been known for a long time [66–70]. It has been proposed that the mechanism for the uptake of these proteins is fluid pinocytosis in the cysticerci of *T. crassiceps* [69]. Moreover, in addition of entering the host proteins, these parasites can also secrete them [70, 71]. The biological role of those uptaken host proteins remains elusive, however, uptake of host albumin has been proposed to be involved in the maintenance of host-parasite osmotic pressure [68] and uptake of host immunoglobulins has been proposed as a mechanism of immune evasion and even as a source of amino acids [72].

Recent quantitative estimates indicated that host proteins might represent 11–13% of the protein content in the vesicular fluid of *T. solium* cysticerci, with albumin and immunoglobulins being the most abundant proteins. The use of high-throughput proteomics, allowed identifying 891 proteins of host origin from a total of 4,259 in a *T. solium* cysticerci whole protein extract [73]; thus, host proteins might represent up to 19% of the total protein species in the larval tissue lysates. Moreover, a fraction of these uptaken host proteins are intact and perhaps functionally active in the tissues of taeniid larvae [71].

6. Utilization of host proteins by cysticerci; iron chaperons and IgG

A known trait of parasitism is the use of the host as a provider of resources; sugars, amino acids, nucleosides, vitamins, coenzymes and/or microelements are good examples of resources that a parasite can acquire from its host. However, considering the abundance and diversity of host proteins present in the tissues of taeniid larvae, a pertinent question would be: are these parasites benefited by the accumulation of host proteins, beyond simply serving as a source of amino acids or as osmotic regulators? We have explored a couple of prospects: the use of host iron chaperones for the management of the parasite's iron necessities, as well as the use of host immunoglobulins as a source of amino acids [70, 71, 74].

Iron is an essential element for virtually all living organisms. Pathogens have evolved mechanisms to uptake iron from their hosts. Usually, iron is uptaken from plasma proteins: hemoglobin (heme prosthetic group) or haptoglobin-hemoglobin complexes, hemopexin (heme prosthetic group), transferrin or lactoferrin (iron), ferritin (iron), etc. In fact, the constant battle between host and pathogens for this element is well-studied [75, 76]. Hepcidin, the hormone that control iron levels in mammals, was first discovered as an antimicrobial peptide [76, 77]. In this light, it is expected that cestodes would acquire iron from their host, however, the mechanism remains elusive. Some evidence have suggested that hemoglobin or the haptoglobin-hemoglobin complexes could serve as an iron source for the cysts [78]. To support this notion, we have documented the immunolocalization of haptoglobin, hemoglobin, hepcidin and ferritin in the cyst; immunoblotting using crude larval extracts confirmed the finding [73]. We also showed that haptoglobin-hemoglobin complexes were detected in crude larval extracts in their expected molecular weight, indicating that those complexes are only marginally degraded. In fact, free haptoglobin purified from cysts protein lysates has been shown to retain their hemoglobin binding activity, suggesting that the cyst are acquiring iron from those sources. However, future studies are needed to understand how the uptake is performed (is there a specific receptor?), how the heme prosthetic group or iron is removed from those complexes? and which parasite proteins are performing those roles.

Another aspect related to the host's protein uptake by tapeworm's larvae, is the utilization of these proteins as a source of amino acids. Internalization of IgG has been traced using a metabolically labeled (Leu-3H) IgG produced *in vitro* using a mice hybridoma [71]. Through *in vitro* culture of *T. crassiceps* (a closely related species of *T. solium*) cysts in the presence of (Leu-3H) mice IgG, uptake of the immunoglobulin can be monitored. Metabolic labelling also allowed tracking incorporation of Leu-3H into newly synthesized cyst proteins. The biochemical analyses revealed that within the tissue extracts, no other radiolabeled proteins were found. The two bands corresponding to the heavy (50 kDa) and light (25 kDa) chains remained intact after 3 days of culture. This would imply that these proteins are negligible used as a source of amino acids for the biosynthesis of the larvae's own proteins. Furthermore, the integrity and functionality of the Igs was conserved, as shown by SDS-PAGE and western blots marked with the Igs purified from tissue extracts. This finding led the research into a new direction: If immunoglobulins (and perhaps other uptaken host proteins) are only a minor source of amino acids [71], what is the fate of uptaken host proteins?

7. The calcareous corpuscles as a final deposit for host proteins

The tracking of metabolically radiolabeled IgG demonstrated that cysticerci do not significantly use these proteins as a major source of amino acids [71]. A possibility was that these proteins could end in the calcareous corpuscles (CC), that are known as a waste of toxic metabolites and other materials. These CC are microscopic calcifications occurring in the lumen of protonephridial canals, resulting after accretion of mineral salts (calcium carbonate and calcium phosphate) on an organic matrix composed by polysaccharides and other macromolecules [79, 80]. The CC

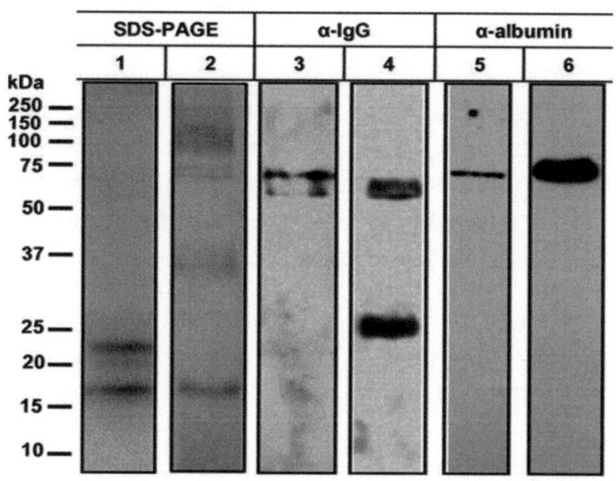

Figure 5.
Immunological identification of host IgG and albumin recovered from the protein matrix of calcareous corpuscles of T. solium *cysticerci. Lanes 1 and 2 correspond to Coomassie blue staining of protein extract from CC and silver staining of porcine serum respectively. Lanes 3 and 5 are western blots of protein extracts obtained from CC, lanes 4 and 6 are gels run with porcine serum, these blots were revealed with an α-IgG coupled to HRP (3 and 4) or sheep α-albumin and then with a rabbit α-sheep IgG coupled to HRP (5 and 6). This figure was originally published in [70].*

are involved in the removal of toxic solutes and regulation of mineral trafficking [81]. Formation of CC has been proposed as a mechanism for protecting cysticerci from calcification [79]. The CC represent about 10% of the dry weight of total larval tissue [82]. It has been estimated that in aged *T. solium* cysticerci, calcareous corpuscles can represent up to 41% of the dry weight [81, 82].

Searching for host proteins in the organic matrix of CC from *T. solium* cysticerci, a mass spectrometry analysis was carried out. A total of 636-760 proteins were identified and quantified, from which 412-508 (60-70%) corresponded to host proteins. *T. solium* proteins in the organic matrix of CC were only 224-252 (30-40%). The remarkable finding that the major protein component in the organic matrix are host proteins, suggests that CC act as a final destination for host proteins. We also showed that intact host proteins can be recovered even after dissolution of CC in a weak acid solution (**Figure 5**). Therefore, these proteins are incorporated into the organic matrix without being degraded [71]. If host antibodies are incorporated into the organic matrix of CC in the form of immune complexes, it is conceivable that cysticerci developed this strategy as a way to diminish exposure of relevant parasite antigens, which could result in a sophisticated mechanism to evade the adaptive humoral immunity of the host.

8. Conclusions

- Genomic and proteomic information on flatworms and particularly on cestode parasites is growing rapidly during the last decade, allowing new approaches to a number of questions.

- Taeniid metacestodes uptake large amounts of host proteins, some of which may be used to meet physiological needs of these parasites.

- Host proteins appear to be marginally degraded; it's importance as a source of amino acids appears to be negligible.

- Proteomic analyses of the organic matrix of the calcareous corpuscles evidenced that a majority of proteins in the organic matrix are of host origin, suggesting that these proteins are sent to the CC as a final destination.

- A consequence of the incremental uptake of host proteins during the lifetime of cysts that terminate being part of the organic matrix of calcareous corpuscles, would be a parallel increment in amount of calcareous corpuscles. Accumulation of corpuscles in larval tissue might represent a biological timer that limits the life span of cysticerci in the host.

Acknowledgements

This report was supported in part by grants A1-5-11306 (CONACYT) and [IN 205820] PAPIIT-UNAM.

Conflict of interest

The authors declare that there are no conflict of interest associated with the manuscript.

Author details

Diana G. Ríos-Valencia[1], José Navarrete-Perea[2], Arturo Calderón-Gallegos[1], Jeannette Flores-Bautista[1] and Juan Pedro Laclette[1*]

1 Biomedical Research Institute, Universidad Nacional Autónoma de México, Mexico City, Mexico

2 Department of Cell Biology, Harvard Medical School, Boston Massachusetts, United States

*Address all correspondence to: laclette@iibiomedicas.unam.mx

References

[1] Webb C, Cabada MM. Intestinal cestodes. Current Opinion in Infectious Diseases 2017;30(5):504-510. DOI: 10.1097/QCO.0b013e3282ef579e

[2] Eckert J, Deplazes P. Biological, Epidemiological, and Clinical Aspects of Echinococcosis, a Zoonosis of Increasing Concern. Clinical Microbiology Reviews. 2004;17(1):107-135. DOI: 10.1128/cmr.17.1.107-135.2004

[3] Gripper LB, Welburn SC. Neurocysticercosis infection and disease–A review. Acta Tropica. 2016; 66:218-224. DOI: 10.1016/j.actatropica.2016.11.015Abba

[4] Abba K, Ramaratnam S, Ranganathan LN. Anthelmintics for people with neurocysticercosis. Cochrane Database of Systematic Reviews 2010;17;2010(3):CD000215. DOI: 10.1002/14651858.CD000215.pub3.

[5] O'Neal SE, Flecker RH. Hospitalization frequency and charges for neurocysticercosis, Emerging Infectious Diseases. 2015;21(6):969-976. DOI:10.3201/eid2106.141324

[6] Brunetti E, Kern P, Vuitton DA. Expert consensus for the diagnosis and treatment of cystic and alveolar echinococcosis in humans. Acta Tropica. 2010;114(1):1-16. DOI: 10.1016/j.actatropica.2009.11.001

[7] Garcia HH, Moro PL, Schantz PM. Zoonotic helminth infections of humans: echinococcosis, cysticercosis and fascioliasis. Current Opinion in Infectious Diseases. 2007;20(5): 489-494. DOI: 10.1097/QCO.0b013e3282a95e39

[8] Olson PD, Littlewood DTJ, Bray RA, Mariaux J. Interrelationships and evolution of the tapeworms (Platyhelminthes: Cestoda). Molecular Phylogenetics and Evolution. 2001;19(3):443-467. DOI: 10.1006/mpev.2001.0930

[9] Egger B. Making Heads or Tails of Tapeworms. Trends in Parasitology. 2016;32(7):511-512. DOI: 10.1016/j.pt.2016.04.003. DOI: 10.1016/j.pt.2016.04.003.

[10] Sulima A, Savijoki K, Bien J, Näreaho A, Salamatin R, Conn DB, et al. Comparative proteomic analysis of *Hymenolepis diminuta* cysticercoid and adult stages. Frontiers in Microbiology. 2018;15;8:2672. DOI:10.3389/fmicb.2017.02672.

[11] Craig P, Ito A. Intestinal cestodes. Current Opinion in Infectious Diseases. 2007;20(5):524-532. DOI: 10.1097/QCO.0b013e3282ef579e

[12] Tsai IJ, Zarowiecki M, Holroyd N, Garciarrubio A, Sanchez-Flores A, Brooks KL, et al. The genomes of four tapeworm species reveal adaptations to parasitism. Nature. 2013;496(7443):57-63. DOI: 10.1038/nature12031

[13] Marzano V, Mancinelli L, Bracaglia G, Del Chierico F, Vernocchi P, Di Girolamo F, et al. "Omic" investigations of protozoa and worms for a deeper understanding of the human gut "parasitome." PLoS Neglected Tropical Diseases. 2017;11(11):e0005916. DOI: 10.1371/journal.pntd.0005916.

[14] Robb SMC, Ross E, Alvarado AS. SmedGD: The *Schmidtea mediterranea* genome database. Nucleic Acids Researcher. 2008;36(SUPPL. 1):D599-D606. DOI:10.1093/nar/gkm684.

[15] Helminth I, Consortium G. Comparative genomics of the major parasitic worms. Nature Genetics. 2019;51(1):163-174. DOI: 10.1038/s41588-018-0262-1.

[16] Zheng H, Zhang W, Zhang L, Zhang Z, Li J, Lu G, et al. The genome of the hydatid tapeworm *Echinococcus granulosus*. Nature. 2013;45(10):1168-1175. DOI:10.1038/ng.2757

[17] Grohme MA, Schloissnig S, Rozanski A, Pippel M, Young GR, Winkler S, et al. The genome of *S. mediterranea* and the evolution of cellular core mechanisms. Nature Publishing Group. 2018;554(7690):56-61. DOI: 10.1038/nature25473.

[18] Rozanski A, Moon HK, Brandl H, Martín-Durán JM, Grohme MA, Hüttner K, et al. PlanMine 3.0 - improvements to a mineable resource of flatworm biology and biodiversity. Nucleic Acids Research. 2019;47(D1):D812–D820. DOI:10.1093/nar/gky1070

[19] Luo F, Yin M, Mo X, Sun C, Wu Q, Zhu B, et al. An improved genome assembly of the fluke *Schistosoma japonicum*. PLoS Neglected Tropical Diseases. 2019;13(8):e0007612. DOI: 10.1371/journal.pntd.0007612

[20] Zhou Y, Zheng H, Chen Y, Zhang L, Wang K, Guo J, et al. The *Schistosoma japonicum* genome reveals features of host-parasite interplay. Nature. 2009; 460(7253):345-351. DOI: 10.1038/nature08140

[21] Young ND, Jex AR, Li B, Liu S, Yang L, Xiong Z, et al. Whole-genome sequence of *Schistosoma haematobium*. Nature Genetics. 2012;44(2):221-225. DOI:10.1038/ng.1065

[22] Stroehlein AJ, Korhonen PK, Chong TM, Lim YL, Chan KG, Webster B, et al. High-quality *Schistosoma haematobium* genome achieved by single-molecule and long-range sequencing. Gigascience. 2019;8(9):1-12. DOI:10.1093/gigascience/giz108

[23] Berriman M, Haas BJ, Loverde PT, Wilson RA, Dillon GP, Cerqueira GC, et al. The genome of the blood fluke *Schistosoma mansoni*. Nature. 2009;460(7253):352-358. DOI: 10.1038/nature08160

[24] Protasio A V., Tsai IJ, Babbage A, Nichol S, Hunt M, Aslett MA, et al. A systematically improved high quality genome and transcriptome of the human blood fluke *Schistosoma mansoni*. PLoS Neglected Tropical Diseases. 2012;6(1):1455. DOI: 10.1371/journal.pntd.0001455

[25] Wang X, Chen W, Huang Y, Sun J, Men J, Liu H, et al. The draft genome of the carcinogenic human liver fluke *Clonorchis sinensis*. Genome Biology. 2011;12(10):R107. DOI: 10.1186/gb-2011-12-10-r107

[26] Huang Y, Chen W, Wang X, Liu H, Chen Y, Guo L, et al. The Carcinogenic Liver Fluke, *Clonorchis sinensis*: New Assembly, Reannotation and Analysis of the Genome and Characterization of Tissue Transcriptomes. PLoS One. 2013;8(1):e54732. DOI: 10.1371/journal.pone.0054732

[27] Wasik K, Gurtowski J, Zhou X, Ramos OM, Delás MJ, Battistoni G, et al. Genome and transcriptome of the regeneration-competent flatworm, *Macrostomum lignano.* PNAS. 2015;112(40):12462-12467. DOI:10.1073/pnas.1516718112

[28] Wudarski J, Simanov D, Ustyantsev K, De Mulder K, Grelling M, Grudniewska M, et al. Efficient transgenesis and annotated genome sequence of the regenerative flatworm model *Macrostomum lignano*. Nature Communications 2017;8(1):1-12. DOI: 10.1038/s41467-017-02214-8

[29] Hahn C, Fromm B, Bachmann L. Comparative Genomics of Flatworms (Platyhelminthes) Reveals Shared Genomic Features of Ecto- and Endoparastic Neodermata. Genome

Biology and Evolution. 2014;6(5):1105-1117. DOI:10.1093/gbe/evu078

[30] Young ND, Nagarajan N, Lin SJ, Korhonen PK, Jex AR, Hall RS, et al. The *Opisthorchis viverrini* genome provides insights into life in the bile duct. Nature Communications. 2014;5(13):1-11. DOI:10.1038/ncomms5378

[31] Wang S, Wang S, Luo Y, Xiao L, Luo X, Gao S, et al. Comparative genomics reveals adaptive evolution of Asian tapeworm in switching to a new intermediate host. Nature Communications. 2016;7(1):1-12. DOI:10.1038/ncomms12845

[32] Maldonado LL, Assis J, Araújo FMG, Salim ACM, Macchiaroli N, Cucher M, et al. The *Echinococcus canadensis* (G7) genome : a key knowledge of parasitic platyhelminth human diseases. BMC Genomics. 2017;1-23. DOI:10.1186/s12864-017-3574-0

[33] McNulty SN, Tort JF, Rinaldi G, Fischer K, Rosa BA, Smircich P, et al. Genomes of Fasciola hepatica from the Americas Reveal Colonization with Neorickettsia Endobacteria Related to the Agents of Potomac Horse and Human Sennetsu Fevers. PLOS Genetics. 2017;13(1):e1006537. DOI:10.1371/journal.pgen.1006537

[34] Li W, Liu B, Yang Y, Ren Y, Wang S, Liu C, et al. The genome of tapeworm *Taenia multiceps* sheds light on understanding parasitic mechanism and control of coenurosis disease. DNA Research. 2018;25(June):499-510. DOI:10.1093/dnares/dsy020

[35] Maldonado LL, Arrabal JP, Rosenzvit MC, Kamenetzky L. Revisiting the Phylogenetic History of Helminths Through Genomics , the Case of the New *Echinococcus oligarthrus* Genome. Frontiers in Genetics. 2019;10:708. DOI:10.3389/fgene.2019.00708

[36] Nowak RM, Jastr JP, Kuśmirek W, Sałamatin R, Rydzanicz M, Sobczyk-kopcioł A, et al. Assembly and annotation of the model tapeworm *Hymenolepis diminuta*. Scientific Data. 2019;3;6(1):302. DOI: 10.1038/s41597-019-0311-3

[37] Ershov NI, Mordvinov VA, Prokhortchouk EB, Pakharukova MY, Gunbin K V., Ustyantsev K, et al. New insights from *Opisthorchis felineus* genome: Update on genomics of the epidemiologically important liver flukes. BMC Genomics 2019;20(1):1-22. DOI: 10.1186/s12864-019-5752-8

[38] Oey H, Zakrzewski M, Narain K, Devi KR, Agatsuma T, Nawaratna S, et al. Whole-genome sequence of the oriental lung fluke *Paragonimus westermani*. Gigascience. 2018; 8(1):1-8. DOI: 10.1093/gigascience/giy146

[39] Oey H, Zakrzewski M, Gravermann K, Young ND, Korhonen PK, Gobert GN, et al. Whole-genome sequence of the bovine blood fluke Schistosoma bovis supports interspecific hybridization with *S. Haematobium*. PLoS Pathogens. 2019;15(1):e1007513–e1007513. DOI: 10.1371/journal.ppat.1007513

[40] Howe KL, Bolt BJ, Shafie M, Kersey P, Berriman M. WormBase ParaSite – a comprehensive resource for helminth genomics. Molecular and Biochemical Parasitology. 2017;215:2-10. DOI: 10.1016/j.molbiopara.2016.11.005

[41] Howe KL, Bolt BJ, Cain S, Chan J, Chen WJ, Davis P, et al. WormBase 2016: expanding to enable helminth genomic research. Nucleic Acids Reseacher. 2016;44(D1):D774–D780. DOI: 10.1093/nar/gkv1217

[42] Thomas SH, Wagner RD, Arakaki AK, Skolnick J, Kirby JR, Shimkets LJ, et al. The Mosaic Genome of *Anaeromyxobacter dehalogenans* Strain 2CP-C Suggests an Aerobic Common

Ancestor to the Delta-Proteobacteria. PLoS One 2008;3(5):e2103. DOI: 10.1371/journal.pone.0002103

[43] Vinogradov AE. Genome size and GC-percent in vertebrates as determined by flow cytometry: The triangular relationship. Cytometry. 1998;31(2):100-109. DOI:10.1002/(sici)1097-0320(19980201)31:2<100::aid-cyto5>3.0.co;2-q

[44] Zhao Z, Zhang F. Sequence context analysis in the mouse genome: Single nucleotide polymorphisms and CpG island sequences. Genomics.;87:68-74. DOI: 10.1016/j.ygeno.2005.09.012

[45] Piovesan A, Pelleri MC, Antonaros F, Strippoli P, Caracausi M, Vitale L. On the length, weight and GC content of the human genome. BMC Research Notes. 2019;12(1):106. DOI:10.1186/s13104-019-4137-z

[46] Riddiford N, Olson PD. Wnt gene loss in flatworms. Development Genes and Evolution. 2011;221(4):187-197. DOI: 10.1007/s00427-011-0370-8

[47] Philippidou P, Dasen JS. Hox Genes: Choreographers in Neural Development, Architects of Circuit Organization. Neuron. 2013;2;80(1):12-34. DOI:10.1016/j.neuron.2013.09.020

[48] Mathers PH, Grinberg A, Mahon KA, Jamrich M. The Rx homeobox gene is essential for vertebrate eye development. Nature. 1997;387(6633):603-607. DOI:10.1038/42475

[49] Castro LFC, Rasmussen SLK, Holland PWH, Holland ND, Holland LZ. A Gbx homeobox gene in amphioxus: Insights into ancestry of the ANTP class and evolution of the midbrain/hindbrain boundary. Developmental Biology. 2006;1;295(1):40-51. DOI: 10.1016/j.ydbio.2006.03.003

[50] Walldorf U, Kiewe A, Wickert M, Ronshaugen M, McGinnis W. Homeobrain, a novel paired-like homeobox gene is expressed in the Drosophila brain. Mechanisms of Development. 2000;96(1):141-144. DOI: 10.1016/s0925-4773(00)00380-4.

[51] Brooke NM, Garcia-Fernàndez J, Holland PWH. The ParaHox gene cluster is an evolutionary sister of the Hox gene cluster. Nature. 1998;15];392(6679):920-2. DOI: 10.1038/31933

[52] Pakharukova MY, Vavilin VA, Sripa B, Laha T, Brindley PJ, Mordvinov VA. Functional Analysis of the Unique Cytochrome P450 of the Liver Fluke Opisthorchis felineus. PLoS Neglected Tropical Diseases. 2015;9(12): e0004258. DOI: doi: 10.1371/journal.pntd.0004258

[53] Salinas G, Selkirk ME, Chalar C, Maizels RM, Fernández C. Linked thioredoxin-glutathione systems in platyhelminths. Trends in Parasitology. 2004, 20(7):340-346. DOI: 10.1016/j.pt.2004.05.002.

[54] Cvilink V, Lamka J, Skálová L. Xenobiotic metabolizing enzymes and metabolism of anthelminthics in helminthes. Drug Metabolism Reviews. 2009; 41(1):8-26. DOI: 10.1080/03602530802602880

[55] Harispe L, García G, Arbildi P, Pascovich L, Chalar C, Zaha A, et al. Biochemical analysis of a recombinant glutathione transferase from the cestode *Echinococcus granulosus*. Acta Tropica. 2010;114(1):31-36. DOI:10.1016/j.actatropica.2009.12.003

[56] Huang X, Xu J, Wang Y, Guo C, Chen L, Gu X, et al. GP50 as a promising early diagnostic antigen for *Taenia multiceps* infection in goats by indirect ELISA. Parasites and Vectors. 2016;9(1):618. DOI: 10.1186/s13071-016-1915-5

[57] Muro C, Gomez-Puerta LA, Flecker RH, Gamboa R, Barreto PV, Dorny P, et al. Porcine cysticercosis: Possible cross-reactivity of *Taenia hydatigena* to GP50 antigen in the enzyme-linked immunoelectrotransfer blot assay. The American Journal of Tropical Medicine and Hygiene. 2017;97(6):1830-1832. DOI: 10.4269/ajtmh.17-0378

[58] Hancock K, Pattabh S, Greene RM, Yushak ML, Williams F,et al. Characterization and cloning of GP50, a *Taenia solium* antigen diagnostic for cysticercosis. Molecular and Biochemical Parasitology. 2004;133(1):115-124. DOI:10.1016/j.molbiopara.2003.10.001

[59] Garcia HH, O'Neal SE, Noh J, Handali S, Gilman RH, Gonzalez AE, et al. Laboratory diagnosis of neurocysticercosis (*Taenia solium*). Journal of Clinical Microbiology. 2018;56(9). DOI: 10.1128/JCM.00424-18

[60] Frayha GJ. Comparative metabolism of acetate in the taeniid tapeworms *Echinococcus granulosus*, *E. multilocularis* and *Taenia hydatigena*. Comparative Biochemistry and Physiology Part B: Comparative Biochemistry Comp Biochem Physiol - Part B Biochem. Elsevier. 1971;39(1):167-170. DOI: 10.1016/0305-0491(71)90264-1

[61] Kanehisa M, Goto S. KEGG: Kyoto Encyclopedia of Genes and Genomes. Nucleic Acids Research, 2000; 1;28(1):27-30. DOI: 10.1093/nar/28.1.27.

[62] Kanehisa M. Toward understanding the origin and evolution of cellular organisms. Protein Science. 2019;28(11):1947-1951. DOI: 10.1002/pro.3715.

[63] Illescas O, Carrero JC, Bobes RJ, Flisser A, Rosas G, Laclette JP. Molecular characterization, functional expression, tissue localization and protective potential of a *Taenia solium* fatty acid-binding protein. Molecular and Biochemical Parasitology. 2012 Dec 1;186(2):117-125. DOI:10.1016/j.molbiopara.2012.10.002

[64] Pearce EJ, Huang SCC. The metabolic control of schistosome egg production. Cell Microbiology. 2015;17(6):796-801. DOI: 10.1111/cmi.12444

[65] Heath RL. Biosynthesis de novo of purines and pyrimidines in *Mesocestoides* (Cestoda) I. International Journal of Parasitology. 1970;56(1):98-102

[66] Hustead ST, Williams JF. Permeability studies on taeniid metacestodes. II. Antibody mediated effects on membrane permeability in larvae of *Taenia taeniaeformis* and *Taenia crassiceps*. Journal of Parasitology. 1977;63(2):322-326

[67] Machnicka B, Grzybowski J. Host serum proteins in *Taenia saginata* metacestode fluid. Veterinary Parasitology. 1986;19(1-2):47-54. DOI:10.1016/0304-4017(86)90031-2

[68] Hayunga EG, Sumner MP, Letonja T. Evidence for selective incorporation of host immunoglobulin by strobilocerci of *Taenia taeniaeformis*. Journal of Parasitology. 1989;75(4):638-642

[69] Ambrosio J, Landa A, Merchant MT, Laclette JP. Protein uptake by cysticerci of *Taenia crassiceps*. Archives of medical research. 1994; 25(3):325-330

[70] Aldridge JR, Jennette MA, Kuhn RE. Uptake and Secretion of Host Proteins by *Taenia crassiceps* Metacestodes. Journal of Parasitology. 2006;1;92(5):1101-2. DOI: 10.1645/GE-835R.1.

[71] Flores-Bautista J, Navarrete-Perea J, Fragoso G, Flisser A, Soberón X,

Laclette JP. Fate of uptaken host proteins in *Taenia solium* and *Taenia crassiceps* cysticerci. Biosciences Report. 2018;6;38(4). DOI: 10.1042/BSR20180636

[72] Damian RT. Presidential Address: The Exploitation of Host Immune Responses by Parasites. Journal of Parasitology. 1987;73(1):1. DOI:10.1017/s0031182097002357

[73] Navarreta-Pera J, Isasa M, Paulo JA, Corral-corral R, Flores-bautista J, Herna B, Gygi SP, et al. Quantitative multiplexed proteomics of *Taenia solium* cysts obtained from the skeletal muscle and central nervous system of pigs. 2017; 25;11(9):e0005962. DOI: 10.1371/journal.pntd.0005962

[74] Navarrete-Perea J, Moguel B, Mendoza-Hernández G, Fragoso G, Sciutto E, Bobes RJ, et al. Identification and quantification of host proteins in the vesicular fluid of porcine *Taenia solium* cysticerci. Experimental Parasitology. 2014 Aug;143(1):11-17. DOI: 10.1016/j.exppara.2014.04.011

[75] Kronstad JW, Caza M. Shared and distinct mechanisms of iron acquisition by bacterial and fungal pathogens of humans. Frontiers in Cellular and Infection Microbiology. 2013; 19;3:80. DOI: 10.3389/fcimb.2013.00080

[76] Barton JC, Acton RT. Hepcidin, iron, and bacterial infection. In: Vitamins and Hormones. Academic Press Inc. 2019;110:223-242. DOI:10.1016/bs.vh.2019.01.011

[77] Yiannikourides A, Latunde-Dada G. A Short Review of Iron Metabolism and Pathophysiology of Iron Disorders. Medicines. 2019;6(3):85. DOI:10.3390/medicines6030085

[78] Navarrete-Perea J, Toledano-Magaña Y, De La Torre P, Sciutto E, Bobes RJ, Soberón X, et al. Role of porcine serum haptoglobin in the host-parasite relationship of *Taenia solium* cysticercosis. Molecular and Biochemical Parasitology. 2016;1;207(2):61-7. DOI: 10.1016/j.molbiopara.2016.05.010

[79] Vargas-Parada L, Merchant MT, Willms K, Laclette JP. Formation of calcareous corpuscles in the lumen of excretory canals of *Taenia solium* cysticerci. Parasitology Research. 1999;85(2):88-92. DOI: 10.1007/s004360050514

[80] von Brand T, Nylen MU, Martin GN, Churchwell FK, Stites E. Cestode calcareous corpuscles: Phosphate relationships, crystallization patterns, and variations in size and shape. Experimental Parasitology. 1969;25(C):291-310. DOI: 10.1016/0014-4894(69)90075-7

[81] McCullough JS, Fairweather I. The structure, composition, formation and possible functions of calcareous corpuscles in *Trilocularia acanthiaevulgaris* Olsson 1867 (Cestoda, Tetraphyllidea). Parasitology Researcher. 1987;74(2):175-182. DOI: 10.1007/BF00536030

[82] Chung YB, Kong Y, Cho SY, Yang HJ. Purification and localization of a 10 kDa calcareous corpuscle binding protein of *Spirometra mansoni* plerocercoid. 2 Parasitology Research. 2003;235-237. DOI: 10.1007/s00436-002-0694-4

Chapter 8

Hormones and Parasites, Their Role in *Taenia solium* and *Taenia crassiceps* Physiology and Development

Marta C. Romano, Ricardo A. Valdez, Martin Patricio, Alejandra Aceves-Ramos, Alex I. Sánchez, Arlet Veloz, Pedro Jiménez and Raúl J. Bobes

Abstract

The host's hormonal environment determines the susceptibility, the course, and severity of several parasite infections. In most cases the infection disturbs the host environment, and activates immune responses that end up affecting the endocrine system. In the other hand, a number of reports indicate that parasites have reproductive systems, and some others have shown that these organisms synthetize sex steroid hormones. We have shown that cysticerci, the larval stage of *Taenia solium and Taenia crassiceps* ORF and WFU, synthesize steroid hormones. This capacity was modified by drugs that act inhibiting the steroid synthesizing enzymes, or blocking the parasite's hormone receptors. We have also shown that the cysticerci of *T. crassiceps* WFU and *T. solium* have the capacity to synthesize corticosteroids as deoxicorticosterone and corticosterone. We also reviewed the effects of insulin on these parasites, and the receptors found for this hormone. A deep knowledge of the parasite's endocrine properties will contribute to understand their reproduction and the reciprocal interactions with the host. Likewise, may also help designing tools to combat the infection in clinical situations.

Keywords: Parasites, *Taenia*, cysticerci, hormones, steroids

1. Introduction

Corticosteroids and sex steroids are crucial in vertebrate reproduction, metabolism and immune response, but their role in invertebrates had received a reduced attention, similarly happen with the influence of peptides and protein hormones in parasite's development. Therefore, we review here the parasite-endocrine system interplays.

The interaction between parasites and the host defines the intensity of parasite infections. In many cases, the presence of parasites in the host changes its endocrine equilibrium due to the activation of the immune system response, which finally affects the host endocrine system through the influence of cytokines and growth factors released by the immune cells. These changes sometimes control the infection, but in many cases the immune system of the host cannot reject the parasite invasion and thereafter the organisms succeed, and rapidly multiply in the host. A role for 17-beta-estradiol in immunoendocrine regulation of murine cysticercosis by *Taenia crassiceps* was verified [1].

Some parasite infections disrupt the host endocrine system, to this regards we recently reported that the chronic infection of female mice with *T. crassiceps* WFU disrupted the ovarian folliculogenesis, causing a significant increase in follicle atresia, and a reduction in the number of corpora lutea (**Figure 1**) [2]. We also showed in that study that *T. crassiceps* cysticerci infection increased the female mice serum estrogen concentrations, an effect that augmented with the infection time, and that the infection increases the ovarian expression of the steroidogenic enzymes P450-aromatase and P450-Cyp19 [2]. We and collaborators also shown that the nervous system infection with *T. solium* cysticerci (neurocysticercosis) caused endocrine alterations in male and female patients [3], and Sacerdote et al. [4] showed that brain cysticerci images reduced or disappeared after treatment with raloxifene in a patient diagnosed with neurocysticecosis.

In some cases, the parasite's infection affects the host reproductive behavior, for example, changes in reproductive behavior occurred in *Taenia crassiceps* ORF infected male mice [5].

1.1 Sex steroids effects

Several reports indicate the host hormonal environment determines the susceptibility, the course, and severity of many parasite infections. Supporting this fact, a clear dichotomy in infection susceptibility between males and females had been observed in some parasitic infections. For example, the rich estrogen environment provided by female mice facilitates *T. crassiceps* ORF cysticerci proliferation [6].

In addition, steroids may directly influence the growth and proliferation of parasites. For example, *T. crassiceps* ORF and WFU cysticerci cell proliferation and metabolism evaluated by ^{3}H-thymidine and MTT incorporation was increased by the addition of physiological concentrations of testosterone, and 17β-estradiol to the culture media [7] and enhance proliferation of *T. crassiceps* ORF cysticerci, a progesterone like receptor was found in these parasites [8].

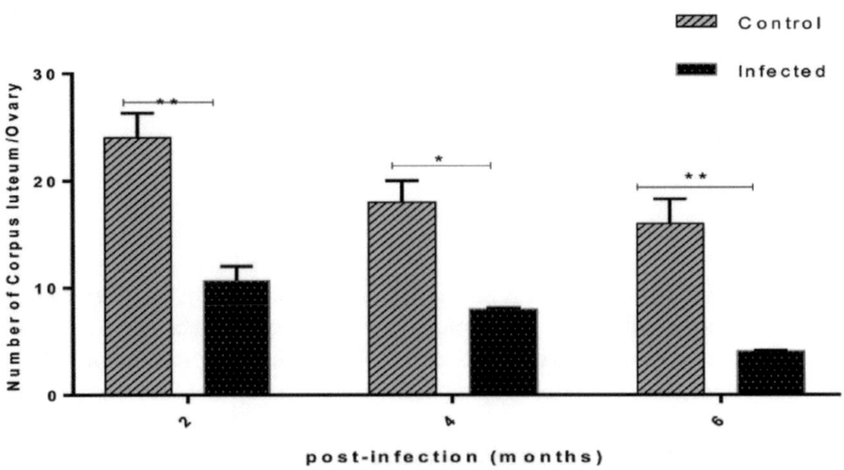

Figure 1.
The infection with Taenia crassiceps *WFU decreased the ovarian corpora lutea of female mice. The number of corpora lutea diminished when the infection progresses.*

Particularly estrogens are important for *T. crassiceps* and *T. solium* cysticerci development. Estrogen synthesis is the result of the transformation of androgens to estrogens by the steroidogenic enzyme P450-Aromatase (Arom) that transforms androstendione and testosterone to the estrogens 17β-estradiol and estrone. Interventions that reduced estrogen synthesis, or affected the binding to its receptors affect the cysticerci proliferation. For instance, the administration of fadrozole, a drug that inhibits Arom, to *T. crassiceps* ORF female infected mice reduced the parasite's load [9].

The presence of steroid receptors in parasites have been documented [10], hence the blockage of steroids receptors might mitigate the effect of these hormones. For example, the expression of an estrogen binding protein similar to nuclear estrogen receptor was shown in *T. crassicpes* ORF cysticerci [11].

Interventions on the sex steroid receptors affect the *T. crassiceps* cysticerci parasite charge. That is the case for the administration of tamoxifen, a competitive antagonist of the estrogen receptor alfa that reduced *in vitro* the proliferation and viability of *T. crassiceps* ORF cysticerci [12] and *in vivo* reduced parasite's load. Likewise, we have shown that the administration of flutamide, an androgen receptor competitor, reduced the parasite proliferation [7].

1.2 Corticosteroids are key hormones in the host-parasite interplay

Corticosteroids are synthesized in the adrenal cortex and are classified as glucocorticoids, mineralocorticoids and adrenal androgens. Cortisol and corticosterone are the main glucocorticoids and are involved in glucose, lipid and protein metabolism. Aldosterone and dexycorticosterone (DOC) are classified as mineralocorticoids because they participate in the hydro-electrolytic balance, whereas adrenal androgens as dehydroepiandrosterone (DHEA) take part in the pubertal process. DHEA is an estrogen precursor that can be transformed to potent androgens in the testis and is an important immune regulator [13].

Cortisol and corticosterone are key hormones in the physiological stress response (in example exercise), and in non-physiological stress situations, such as social isolation, persecution, infections, etc., all circumstances that increase serum corticosteroids levels. It is now generally accepted that prolonged stress conducts to impairment of the immune response.

1.2.1 Corticosteroid use in neurocysticercosis

Corticosteroids are employed to prevent or modulate the brain inflammation that follows anthelmintic treatment of parasitic cysts with cysticidal drugs as albendazole or praziquantel [14–16]. The absence of corticosteroids administration in the cysticidal treatment initiates an acute immune response to the parasite that conducts to serious clinical symptoms as seizures, brain edema, and death. These side effects are caused by neuroinflammation and are effectively managed with corticosteroids. On the other side, the administration of dexamethasone plus albendazol to Balb/c mice reduced the cysticidal effect of albendazole [17].

1.2.2 In vitro *effects of glucocorticoids on parasite growth and viability*

It had been shown that corticosteroids may directly influence parasite's proliferation and metabolism. For instance, we had shown that corticosterone and dexamethasone increase the capacity of *T. crassiceps* WFU cysticerci to synthesize androgens and estrogens, hormones that favor the parasite reproduction [18].

1.3 *Taenia solium* and *crassicpes* synthesize steroid hormones

1.3.1 Sex steroids and corticosteroids

The adult worm of *T. solium* and *T. crassiceps* WFU remain attached to the host gut with hooks placed in their head, and develop reproductive units called proglottids, where testis and ovaries gradually differentiate, and finally contain spermatocytes and infective eggs [19]. As stated elsewhere *T. solium* cysticerci is the larval stage of the parasite and is found in the brain or muscle of humans and pigs, whereas *T. crassiceps* WFU cysticerci constitute a useful laboratory model due to their reproduction by budding in the peritoneal cavity of mice. In the last years we have been investigating if *T. solium* and *T. crassiceps* ORF and WFU cysticerci and tapeworms synthesize sex steroids *in vitro.* We found that *T. solium* and *T. crassiceps* ORF cysticerci transform steroid precursors such as progesterone, DHEA, and androstenedione to androgens and estrogens, the capacity to transform precursors to testosterone was related to the developmental stage of the larvae (**Table 1**) [20–22]. These findings demonstrated that *Taenids* are steroidogenic organisms.

Our group have also examined the capacity of *T. solium* and *T. crassiceps* WFU to synthesize corticosteroids. Thereafter, we had incubated *T. crassiceps* cysticerci in the presence of ^{3}H-progesterone and found an important transformation into DOC, a steroid that has mineralocorticoid functions in vertebrates [23, 24]. The addition to the culture medium of metyrapone, a drug used for the medical control of hypercortisolism in Cushing's syndrome, reduced the cysticerci corticosteroid synthesis [23]. In addition, the parasites synthesized corticosterone, which was measured by radioimmunoassay in the culture media. More recently, we found corticosteroid-like synthesis in *T. solium* and *T. crassiceps* tapeworms [24, 25]. To note, the steroidogenic capacity of *T. crassiceps* is related to the development of the parasite [24]. Besides their effects on the own parasite development and differentiation, the cysticerci and tapeworm's steroidogenic capacity might play a role in the permanence of the parasites in the host tissues and organs, by disturbing the host immune cell response.

1.3.2 Taenia solium *and* Taenia crassiceps *and steroidogenic enzymes. Repurposed drugs affect the capacity of parasites to synthesize hormones*

Tritiated androstenediol and testosterone were recovered from the culture media of *T. crassiceps* incubated with ^{3}H-DHEA indicating the presence and activity of enzymes from the Δ5 steroid pathway in these tapeworms [26].

The effect of enzyme inhibitors on the steroid synthesis by *T. crassiceps* WFU cysticerci was investigated by [27]. This study demonstrated that fadrozole, a drug that inhibits P450-aromatase, reduced the transformation of 3H-androstenedione to 17β-estradiol (**Figure 2**), while danazol that inhibits 3β-hydroxysteroid dehydrogenase and 17β-hydroxisteroid dehydrogenase, reduced the transformation of 3H-DHEA to androstendiol, testosterone and 17βestradiol. The incubation of cysticerci with tritiated progesterone as a precursor and different concentrations of ketoconazole that inhibits 11β-hydroxilase, 17α-hydroxilase and 17-20 lyase, resulted in the reduction of the synthesis of tritiated 3H-DOC [27].

We have recently shown that *Taenia solium* cysticerci express the enzyme 17β-HSD that belongs to the short chain dehydrogenases/reductase family [28]. Transient transfection of HEK293T cells with Tsol17β-HSD-pcDNA3.1 (+) induced expression of Tsol17β-HSD that transformed ^{3}H-androstenedione into testosterone (**Figure 3**). In contrast, ^{3}H-estrone was not significantly transformed into estradiol. Therefore, *T. solium* cysticerci express a 17β-HSD that catalyzes the androgen reduction and belongs to the short chain dehydrogenases/reductase (SDR) protein

Radioactive precursor metaboliteS	Transformation rate evaluated in two developmental stages of *Taenia crassiceps* WFU cysticerci	
^{3}H-A$_4$/Testosterone	Invaginated cysticerci	Evaginated cysticerci
6 hours	9.6 ± 2.1	22.9 ± 1.9**
24 hours	71.4 ± 7.6	75.5 ± 4.5
43 hours	75.0 ± 4.7	74.1 ± 5.3
^{3}H-A$_4$/Estradiol		
6 hours	7.7 ± 2.7	5.3 ± 3.3
24 hours	4.7 ± 2.7	3.8 ± 4.3
43 hours	3.1 ± 2.5	0.1 ± 0.5

$^{**}p < 0.01$.

Table 1.
Synthesis of sex steroids by Taenia crassiceps *WFU cysticerci. The parasites were incubated by different periods in the presence of ^{3}H-androstenedione, the culture media was analyzed by TLC. The synthesized steroids are express as percent transformation of the tritiated precursor.*

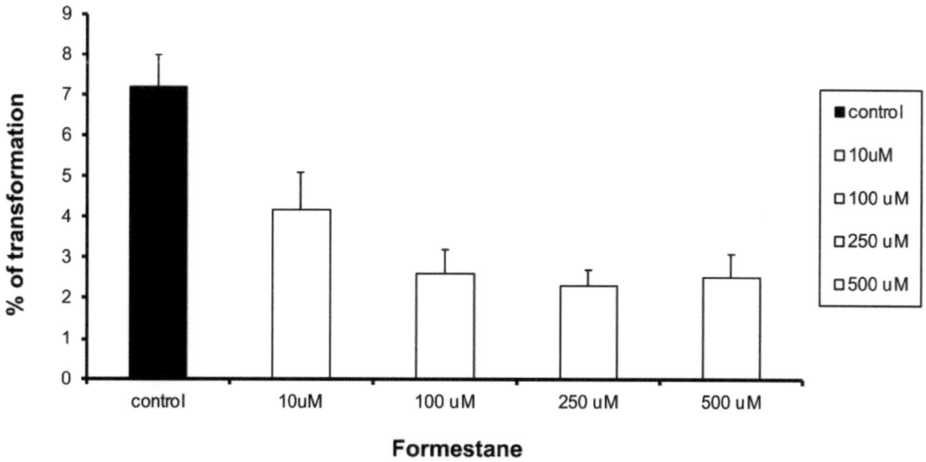

Figure 2.
Effect of formestane, an inhibitor of P450-aromatase, on the synthesis of 17β-estradiol by T. Crassiceps *WFU cysticerci. The parasites were incubated with ^{3}H-androstenedione for 24 h. The percent of tritiated 17β-estradiol synthesized was determined by TLC.*

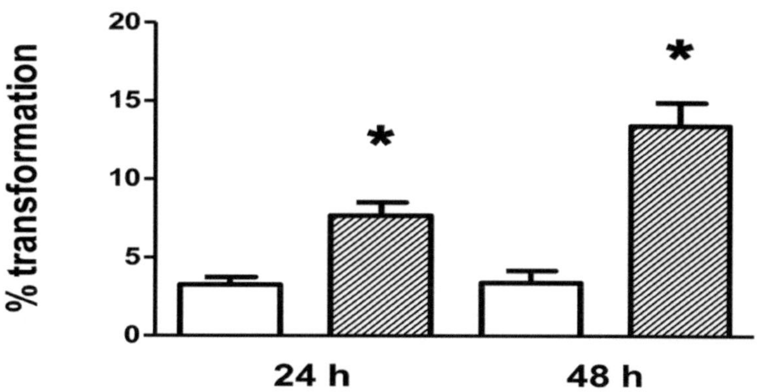

Figure 3.
Testosterone production by HEK293T cells transfected with Tsol-17βHSD-pcDNA3.1(+). After 24 h of transfection with Tsol-17βHSD-pcDNA3.1(+) (white bars) or with pcDNA3.1(+) (black bars), cells were incubated with ^{3}H-androstenedioned for 24 or 48 h. The percent of tritiated testosterone was determined by TLC.

superfamily [28]. A sequence with an identity of 84% with Tsol-17βHSD and a total coverage has been described for *E. multilocularis*, suggesting the presence of 17β-HSD enzymes in these parasites [29]. However, the expression level and enzyme activity of this species has not been yet investigated.

1.4 Additional hormones studied in *T. solium* and *Taenia crassiceps*

Insulin is a potent metabolic hormone that exerts a wide variety of effects. The main metabolic effect of insulin is to stimulate glucose uptake and utilization in muscle and fat tissue, but this hormone also increases lipogenesis, and even acts on protein synthesis. Insulin signaling through insulin receptors (IR) is an ancient and well conserved pathway in metazoan cells organized as transmembrane proteins with tyrosine kinase activity. To note, the uptake and metabolism of glucose is crucial for *T. solium* and *crassiceps* survival.

We have shown that incubation of *T. crassiceps* cysticerci with insulin increased the reproduction of the parasites and also found that female mice exposed to insulin had larger parasite loads than control mice inoculated with vehicle [30]. In the same study an insulin-like receptor present in *T. solium* and *T. crassiceps* was amplified by reverse transcriptase-polymerase chain reaction.

Using genome-wide screening Wang et al. [31] identified putative insulin-like peptides in several parasitic platyhelmths as *T. solium*. Furthermore, two insulin receptor genes were identified and characterized in *T. solium*. The receptors were found in diverse zones of the parasite and are involved in the uptake of glucose, that is crucial for these parasites [32].

The effect of human chorionic gonadotropin (hCG) on the growth and proliferation of larval stages of *T. crassiceps* (WFU strain) and *T. solium*, and the presence of receptors for this hormone in different developmental phases of both cultured parasites was reported [33, 34].

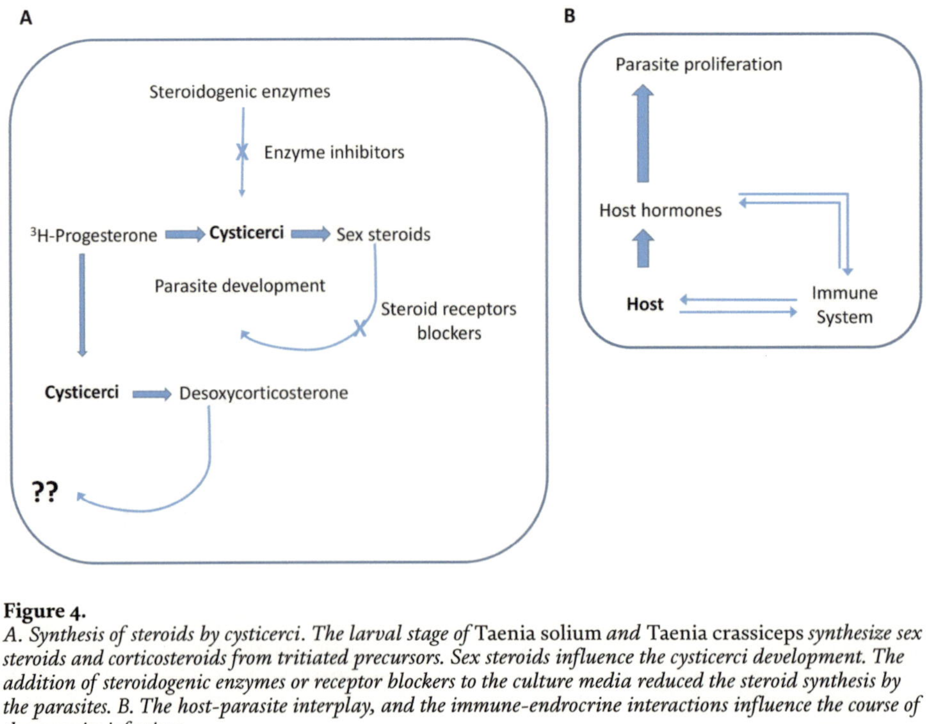

Figure 4.
A. Synthesis of steroids by cysticerci. The larval stage of Taenia solium *and* Taenia crassiceps *synthesize sex steroids and corticosteroids from tritiated precursors. Sex steroids influence the cysticerci development. The addition of steroidogenic enzymes or receptor blockers to the culture media reduced the steroid synthesis by the parasites. B. The host-parasite interplay, and the immune-endrocrine interactions influence the course of the parasite infections.*

2. Conclusions

The interaction between parasites and the host defines the intensity of parasite infections. Steroid hormones play an important role in this interplay. Sex steroids and corticosteroids modify *in vitro* the proliferation of *T. solium* and *T. crassiceps* ORF and WFU cysticerci. Cysticerci and worms have the capacity to synthesize corticosteroids and sex steroids from tritiated precursors, a fact that suggested they have several active steroidogenic enzymes. One of these enzymes, 17β-hydroxysteroid dehydrogenase like was characterized and cloned in *T. solium* cysticerci. The steroidogenic capacity of these parasites was modified with repurposed drugs that affects steroidogenic enzymes as formestane that acts on P450-aromatase, danazol and ketoconazol (**Figure 4**). Insulin modifies the proliferation of cysticerci, and receptors for insulin had been found in parasites. Steroidogenic enzymes inhibitors, and receptors blockers might be used as therapeutic tools for the control of parasitic infections

Acknowledgements

Thanks to Rangel-Rivera Omar for his technical contribution with Figures and Table.

Conflict of interest

The authors declare that they have no known conflict of interests or personal relationships that could have appeared to influence the work reported in this chapter.

Author details

Marta C. Romano[1*], Ricardo A. Valdez[1], Martin Patricio[1], Alejandra Aceves-Ramos[1], Alex I. Sánchez[1], Arlet Veloz[1], Pedro Jiménez[1] and Raúl J. Bobes[2*]

1 Department of Biophysical Physiology and Neurosciences, CINVESTAV del I.P.N, Ciudad de México, Mexico

2 Immunology Department, Biomedical Research Institute, Universidad Nacional Autónoma de México, Ciudad de México, Mexico

*Address all correspondence to: mromano@fisio.cinvestav.mx and rbobes@iibiomedicas.unam.mx

References

[1] Terrazas LI, Bojalil R, Govezensky T, Larralde CJ. A role for 17-beta-estradiol in immunoendocrine regulation of murine cysticercosis (*Taenia crassiceps*). J Parasitol. 1994;80: 563-568. DOI: org/10.2307/3283192

[2] Veloz A, Reyes-Vázquez L, Patricio-Gómez JM, Romano MC. Effect of mice *Taenia crassiceps* WFU cysticerci infection on the ovarian folliculogenesis, enzyme expression, and serum estradiol. Exp Parasitol. 2019;207:107778. DOI: 10.1016/j.exppara.2019.107778

[3] Cárdenas G, Valdez RA, Sáenz B, Bottasso A, Fragoso G, Sciutto E, Romano MC, Fleury A. Impact of *Taenia solium* neurocysticercosis upon endocrine status and its relation with immuno-inflammatory parameters. Int. J. Parasitol. 2012;42:171-176. DOI: 10.1016/j.ijpara.2011.11.009

[4] Sacerdote AS, Mejía JO, Bahtiyar G, Salamon O. Effect of raloxifene in human neurocysticercosis. BMJ Case Rep. 2012;14: bcr0620114417. DOI: 10.1136/bcr.06.2011.4417

[5] Morales J, Larralde C, Arteaga M, Govezensky T, Romano MC, Moralí G. Inhibition of sexual behavior in male mice infected with *Taenia crassiceps* cysticerci. J. Parasitol. 1996;82:689-693. DOI: org/10.2307/3283875

[6] Larralde C, Sciutto E, Huerta L, Terrazas I, Fragoso G, Trueba L, Lemus D, Lomelí C, Tapia G, Montoya RM, et al. Experimental cysticercosis by *Taenia crassiceps* in mice: factors involved in susceptibility. Acta Leiden. 1989;57(2):131-134. PMID: 2488991

[7] Romano MC, Valdez RA, Cartas AL, Gómez Y, Larralde C. Steroid hormone production by parasites: the case of *Taenia crassiceps* and *Taenia solium* cysticerci. J. Steroid Biochem. Mol. Biol. 2003;85:221-225. DOI: 10.1016/S0960-0760(03)00233-4

[8] Aguilar-Díaz H, Nava-Castro KE, Escobedo G, Domínguez-Ramírez L, García-Varela M, Del Río-Araiza VH, Palacios-Arreola MI, Morales-Montor J. A novel progesterone receptor membrane component (PGRMC) in the human and swine parasite *Taenia solium*: implications to the host-parasite relationship. Parasit Vectors. 2018;11(1): 161. DOI: 10.1186/s13071-018-2703-1

[9] Morales-Montor J, Hallal-Caballeros C, Romano MC, Damian R T. Inhibition of P450-aromatase prevents feminization and induces protection during cisticercosis. Int. J. Parasitol. 2002;32:1379-1387. DOI: 10.1016/S0020-7519(02)00130-3

[10] Wu W, LoVerde PT. Nuclear hormone receptors in parasitic helminths. Mol Cell Endocrinol. 2011;334(1-2):56-66. DOI: 10.1016/j.mce.2010.06.011

[11] Ibarra-Coronado EG, Escobedo G, Nava-Castro K, Jesús Ramses CR, Hernández-Bello R, García-Varela M, Ambrosio JR, Reynoso-Ducoing O, Fonseca-Liñán R, Ortega-Pierres G, Pavón L, Hernández ME, Morales Montor J. A helminth cestode parasite express an estrogen-binding protein resembling a classic nuclear estrogen receptor. Steroids. 2011;76(10-11):1149-1159. DOI: 10.1016/j.steroids.2011.05.003

[12] Vargas-Villavicencio JA, Larralde C, De León-Nava MA, Escobedo G, Morales-Montor J. Tamoxifen treatment induces protection in murine cysticercosis. J Parasitol. 2007;93(6): 1512-1517. DOI: 10.1645/GE-1191.1

[13] Romano MC, Pedernera Romano C. Glándulas suprarenales. In: Fisiología

Humana. J. A.F. Tresguerres et al. Mc Graw Hill, 4th ed. Cap. 76. Pag.939-950. ISBN: 978-607-15-0349-7

[14] Nash TE, Mahanty S, Garcia HH, Cysticercosis Group in Peru. Corticosteroid use in neurocysticercosis. Expert Rev Neurother. 2013;11:1175-83. DOI: 10.1586/ern.11.86

[15] Webb CM, White AC Jr. Update on the diagnosis and management of neurocysticercosis. Curr Infect Dis Rep. 2016;18:44. DOI: 10.1007/s11908-016-0547-4

[16] White AC, Coyle CM, Rajshekhar V, Singh G, Hauser WA, Mohanty A, et al. Diagnosis and treatment of neurocysticercosis: 2017 clinical practice guidelines by the Infectious Diseases Society of America (IDSA) and the American Society of Tropical Medicine and Hygiene (ASTMH). Am J Trop Med Hyg. 2018;98:945-966. DOI: 10.4269/ajtmh.18-88751

[17] Palomares-Alonso F, Toledo A, Palencia Hernández G, Jung-Cook H, Fleury A. Effect of dexamethasone on albendazole cysticidal activity in experimental cysticercosis by *Taenia crassiceps* in BALB/c mice: *In vitro* and *in vivo* evaluation. Exp Parasitol. 2020;208:107801. DOI: 10.1016/j.exppara.2019.107801

[18] Hinojosa L, Valdez RA, Salvador V, Rodriguez AG, Willms K, Romano MC. The effect of corticosteroids on sex steroid synthesis in cultured *Taenia crassiceps* Wake Forest University (WFU) cysticerci. J. Helminthol. 2011;86:465-469. DOI: 10.1017/S0022149X11000708

[19] Willms K, Caro JA, Robert L. Ultrastructure of spermatogonia and spermatocyte lobules in *Taenia solium* strobilac (Cestoda, *Cyclophyllidea, Taeniidae*) from golden hamsters. Parasitol. Res. 2003;90:479-488. DOI: 10.1007/s00436-003-0897-3

[20] Gómez Y, Valdez RA, Larralde C, Romano MC. Sex steroids and parasitism. *Taenia crassiceps* cysticercus metabolizes exogenous androstenedione to testosterone *in vitro*. J. Steroid. Biochem. Mol. Biol. 2000;74:143-147. DOI: 10.1016/S0960-0760(00)00099-6

[21] Jiménez P, Valdéz RA, Romano MC. Metabolism of steroid hormones by *Taenia solium* and *Taenia crassiceps* cysticerci. J. Steroid Biochem. Mol. 2006;99:203-208. DOI: 10.1016/j.jsbmb.2006.01.002

[22] Valdez RA, Jiménez P, Cartas AL, Gómez Y, Romano MC. *Taenia solium* cysticerci synthesize androgens and estrogens *in vitro*. Parasitol. Res. 2006; 98:472-476. DOI: 10.1007/s00436-005-0095-6

[23] Valdez RA, Hinojosa L, Gómez Y, Willms K, Romano MC. *Taenia crassiceps* WFU cysticerci synthesize corticosteroids *in vitro*: metyrapone regulates the production. Comp. Endocrinol. 2012;176:409-414. DOI: 10.1016/j.ygcen.2012.01.015

[24] Patricio-Gómez JM, Valdez RA, Veloz A, Aguilar-Vega L, Zurabian R, Romano MC. The synthesis of steroids by *Taenia crassiceps* WFU cysticerci and tapeworms is related to the developmental stages of the parasites. Gen Comp Endocrinol. 2018;259:154-160. DOI: 10.1016/j.ygcen.2017.11.018

[25] Valdez RA, Jiménez P, Fernández-Presas AM, Aguilar L, Willms K, Romano MC. *Taenia solium* tapeworms synthesize corticosteroids and sex steroids *in vitro*. Gen. Comp. Endocrinol. 2014;205:62-67. DOI: 10.1016/j.ygcen.2014.04.014

[26] Fernández Presas AM, Willms K, Romano MC. The key steroidogenic enzyme 3ß-hydroxysteroid dehydrogenase is present in the strobilae and larvae of *Taenia solium* and *T. crassiceps* WFU strain. Parasitol. Res.

2008;103:847-852. DOI: 10.1007/s00436-008-1066-5

[27] Aceves-Ramos A, Valdez RA, Gaona B, Willms K, Romano MC. Steroid synthesis by *Taenia crassiceps* WFU cysticerci is regulated by enzyme inhibitors. Gen. Comp. Endocrinol. 2013;188:212-217. DOI: 10.1016/j.ygcen.2013.03.034

[28] Aceves-Ramos A, de la Torre P, Hinojosa L, Ponce A, García-Villegas R, Laclette JP, Bobes RJ, Romano MC. Cloning, characterization and functional expression of *Taenia solium* 17 beta-hydroxysteroid dehydrogenase. Gen Comp Endocrinol. 2014;203:186-192. DOI: 10.1016/j.ygcen.2014.03.021

[29] Tsai I. J., Zarowiecki M., Holroyd N., Garciarrubio A., Sanchez-Flores A., Brooks K. L., et al. The genomes of four tapeworm species reveal adaptations to parasitism. Nature 2013;496: 57-63. DOI: 10.1038/nature12031

[30] Escobedo G, Romano MC, Morales-Montor J. Differential in vitro effects of insulin on *Taenia crassiceps* and *Taenia solium* cysticerci. J Helminthol. 2009;83(4):403-12. DOI: 10.1017/S0022149X09990265

[31] Wang S, Luo X, Zhang S, Yin C, Dou Y, Cai X. Identification of putative insulin-like peptides and components of insulin signaling pathways in parasitic platyhelminths by the use of genome-wide screening. FEBS J. 2014;281(3): 877-93. DOI: 10.1111/febs.12655

[32] Wang L, Liang P, Wei Y, Zhang S, Guo A, Liu G, Ehsan M, Liu M, Luo X. *Taenia solium* insulin receptors: promising candidates for cysticercosis treatment and prevention. Acta Trop. 2020;209:105552. DOI: 10.1016/j.actatropica.2020.105552

[33] Díaz-Orea MA, de Aluja AS, Erosa ML, Gomez-Conde E, Castellanos Sánchez VO, Willms K, Sciutto E, Fragoso G. Different effects of chorionic gonadotropin on *Taenia crassiceps* and *Taenia solium* cysticerci cultured *in vitro*. J Parasitol. 2007;93(6):1518-1520. DOI: 10.1645/GE-1196.1

[34] Castellanos-Sánchez VO, Gómez-Conde E, Rocha-Gracia RC, Pimentel A, Aluja A, Hernández-Jáuregui P, Huerta M, Díaz-Orea MA. Chorionic gonadotropin hormone receptors on *Taenia solium* and *Taenia crassiceps* cysticerci in culture. J Parasitol. 2009;95(6):1287-1294. DOI: 10.1645/GE-2087.1